Local and Regional Flaps of the Head and Neck

Editors

DIN LAM
ROBERT A. STRAUSS

ORAL AND MAXILLOFACIAL SURGERY CLINICS OF NORTH AMERICA

www.oralmaxsurgery.theclinics.com

Consulting Editor
RICHARD H. HAUG

August 2014 • Volume 26 • Number 3

ELSEVIER

1600 John F. Kennedy Boulevard • Suite 1800 • Philadelphia, Pennsylvania, 19103-2899

http://www.oralmaxsurgery.theclinics.com

ORAL AND MAXILLOFACIAL SURGERY CLINICS OF NORTH AMERICA Volume 26, Number 3
August 2014 ISSN 1042-3699, ISBN-13: 978-0-323-32020-7

Editor: John Vassallo; j.vassallo@elsevier.com
Developmental Editor: Yonah Korngold

Oral and Maxillofacial Surgery Clinics of North America (ISSN 1042-3699) is published quarterly by Elsevier Inc., 360 Park Avenue South, New York, NY 10010-1710. Months of issue are February, May, August, and November. Business and Editorial Offices: 1600 John F. Kennedy Blvd., Suite 1800, Philadelphia, PA 19103-2899. Periodicals postage paid at New York, NY and additional mailing offices. Subscription prices are $385.00 per year for US individuals, $567.00 per year for US institutions, $175.00 per year for US students and residents, $455.00 per year for Canadian individuals, $680.00 per year for Canadian institutions, $520.00 per year for international individuals, $680.00 per year for international institutions and $235.00 per year for Canadian and foreign students/residents. To receive student/resident rate, orders must be accompanied by name or affiliated institution, date of term, and the *signature* of program/residency coordinator on institution letterhead. Orders will be billed at individual rate until proof of status is received. Foreign air speed delivery is included in all *Clinics* subscription prices. All prices are subject to change without notice. **POSTMASTER:** Send address changes to *Oral and Maxillofacial Surgery Clinics of North America,* Elsevier Periodicals Customer Service, 11830 Westline Industrial Drive, St. Louis, MO 63146. Tel: 1-800-654-2452 (U.S. and Canada); 314-447-8871 (outside U.S. and Canada). Fax: 314-447-8029. E-mail: journalscustomerservice-usa@elsevier.com (for print support); journalsonlinesupport-usa@elsevier.com (for online support).

Reprints. For copies of 100 or more, of articles in this publication, please contact the Commercial Reprints Department, Elsevier Inc., 360 Park Avenue South, New York, NY 10010-1710. Tel.: 212-633-3874; Fax: 212-633-3820; Email: reprints@elsevier.com.

Oral and Maxillofacial Surgery Clinics of North America is covered in *MEDLINE/PubMed* (*Index Medicus*), *Science Citation Index Expanded* (*SciSearch®*), *Journal Citation Reports/Science Edition*, and *Current Contents®/Clinical Medicine*.

Contributors

CONSULTING EDITOR

RICHARD H. HAUG, DDS
Carolinas Center for Oral Health, Charlotte,
North Carolina

EDITORS

DIN LAM, DMD, MD
Formerly, Clinical Assistant Professor,
Department of Oral and Facial Surgery,
Virginia Commonwealth University Medical
Center, Richmond, Virginia

ROBERT A. STRAUSS, DDS, MD
Professor of Surgery; Director of Residency
Training Program, Department of Oral and
Facial Surgery, Virginia Commonwealth
University Medical Center, Richmond, Virginia

AUTHORS

XENA ALAKAILY, DDS
Research Fellow, Department of Oral and
Maxillofacial Surgery, Case Western Reserve
University, Cleveland, Ohio

JONATHAN S. BAILEY, DMD, MD, FACS
Clinical Associate Professor, Department
of Surgery, University of Illinois Urbana-
Champaign College of Medicine; Residency
Program Director, Division of Oral and
Maxillofacial Surgery; Division of Head and
Neck Cancer, Carle Foundation Hospital,
Urbana, Illinois

DALE A. BAUR, DDS, MD
Associate Professor and Chair,
Department of Oral and Maxillofacial
Surgery, University Hospitals of Cleveland,
Case Western Reserve University,
Cleveland, Ohio

TUAN BUI, MD, DMD
Department of Oral, Head and Neck Oncology,
Providence Portland Cancer Center; Oral and
Maxillofacial Surgery, Legacy Emanuel
Medical Center; Affiliate Assistant Professor of
Oral and Maxillofacial Surgery, Oregon Health
Sciences University; Head and Neck Surgical
Associates, Portland, Oregon

DANIEL CAMERON BRAASCH, DMD
Former Chief Resident, Department of Oral
and Facial Surgery, Virginia Commonwealth
University Medical Center, Richmond, Virginia

ERIC R. CARLSON, DMD, MD, FACS
Professor and Kelly L. Krahwinkel Chairman;
Director of Oral and Maxillofacial Surgery
Residency Program; Director of Oral/Head and
Neck Oncologic Surgery Fellowship Program;
Department of Oral and Maxillofacial Surgery,
University of Tennessee Medical Center,
University of Tennessee Cancer Institute,
Knoxville, Tennessee

ALLEN CHENG, DDS, MD
Fellow, Head and Neck Oncology, Providence
Portland Cancer Center; Oral and Maxillofacial
Surgery, Legacy Emanuel Medical Center;
Department of Oral and Maxillofacial Surgery,
Oregon Health Sciences University, Portland,
Oregon

KELLY CUNNINGHAM, MD
Clinical Associate Professor, Department
of Surgery, University of Illinois Urbana-
Champaign College of Medicine; Division
of Head and Neck Cancer; Division of
Otolaryngology, Carle Foundation Hospital,
Urbana, Illinois

JASJIT DILLON, DDS, MBBS, FDSRCS, FACS
Program Director, Assistant Clinical Professor, Department of Oral and Maxillofacial Surgery, University of Washington, Seattle, Washington

RUI P. FERNANDES, DMD, MD
Associate Professor, Department of Oral and Maxillofacial Surgery, College of Medicine, University of Florida; Division of Surgical Oncology, Department of Surgery, College of Medicine, University of Florida, Jacksonville, Florida

JASON A. JAMALI, DDS, MD
Clinical Assistant Professor, Department of Oral and Maxillofacial Surgery, University of Illinois at Chicago, Chicago, Illinois

TONG JI, DDS, MD, PhD
Department of Oral Maxillofacial-Head and Neck Oncology, Shanghai Ninth People's Hospital, Shanghai Jiao Tong University, Shanghai, China

DEEPAK KADEMANI, DMD, MD, FACS
Medical Director, Department of Oral and Maxillofacial Surgery; Fellowship Director, Oral/Head and Neck Oncologic Surgery, North Memorial Medical Center and Hubert Humphrey Cancer Center; Associate Professor, Oral and Maxillofacial Surgery, University of Minnesota, Minneapolis, Minnesota

NICHOLAS J. KAIN, DDS
Chief Resident, Department of Oral and Facial Surgery, Virginia Commonwealth University Medical Center, Richmond, Virginia

D. DAVID KIM, DMD, MD
Associate Professor, Department of Oral and Maxillofacial Surgery/Head and Neck Surgery, Louisiana State University Health Sciences Center, Shreveport, Louisiana

DIN LAM, DMD, MD
Formerly, Clinical Assistant Professor, Department of Oral and Facial Surgery, Virginia Commonwealth University Medical Center, Richmond, Virginia

DIANA JEE-HYUN LYU, DDS
Resident, Division of Oral and Maxillofacial Surgery, University of Minnesota, Minneapolis, Minnesota

MEHDI B. MATIN, DDS
Resident, Department of Oral and Maxillofacial Surgery, University of Washington, Seattle, Washington

ESTHER S. OH, DDS, MD
Assistant Professor, Department of Oral and Maxillofacial Surgery, University of Florida at Gainesville, Gainesville, Florida

HUI SHAN ONG, BDS, MD
Department of Oral Maxillofacial-Head and Neck Oncology, Shanghai Ninth People's Hospital, Shanghai Jiao Tong University, Shanghai, China

KETAN PATEL, DDS, PhD
Fellow, Oral/Head and Neck Oncologic Surgery, Department of Oral and Maxillofacial Surgery, North Memorial Medical Center and Hubert Humphrey Cancer Center, Minneapolis, Minnesota

CARLOS A. RAMIREZ, DDS, MD
Division of Oral and Maxillofacial Surgery, Center for Head and Neck, Maxillofacial and Reconstructive Surgery, St. John Providence Health System, Warren, Michigan

ANASTASIOS SAKELLARIOU, DMD, MD
Resident, Oral and Maxillofacial Surgery Department, Boston University, Boston, Massachusetts

ANDREW SALAMA, DDS, MD, FACS
Associate Professor, Program Director, Oral and Maxillofacial Surgery Department, Boston University, Boston, Massachusetts

TODD A. SCHULTZ, DMD
Department of Surgery, University of Illinois Urbana-Champaign College of Medicine; Division of Oral and Maxillofacial Surgery, Carle Foundation Hospital, Urbana, Illinois

RYAN J. SMART, DMD, MD
Fellow, Department of Oral and Maxillofacial Surgery/Head and Neck Surgery, Louisiana State University Health Sciences Center, Shreveport, Louisiana

ROBERT A. STRAUSS, DDS, MD
Professor of Surgery; Director of Residency Training Program, Department of Oral and Facial Surgery, Virginia Commonwealth University Medical Center, Richmond, Virginia

JONATHAN WILLIAMS, DMD, MD
Former Chief Resident, Department of Oral
and Maxillofacial Surgery, University
Hospitals of Cleveland, Case Western
Reserve University, Cleveland, Ohio

MELVYN S. YEOH, DMD, MD
Assistant Professor, Department of Oral and
Maxillofacial Surgery/Head and Neck Surgery,
Louisiana State University Health Sciences
Center, Shreveport, Louisiana

CHEN PING ZHANG, DDS, MD, PhD
Department of Oral Maxillofacial-Head and
Neck Oncology, Shanghai Ninth People's
Hospital, Shanghai Jiao Tong University,
Shanghai, China

Contents

> Basic flap design utilization for reconstruction of head and neck defects requires creativity from the surgeon. Ultimately, the surgeon must closely restore the basic functions and properties of the surgical flap and adjacent tissue. All options within the reconstructive ladder should be considered. When possible, like should be replaced with like (similar tissue) within an esthetic zone. When considering a flap design, the surgeon must remember that the donor site must be closed in an esthetic and functional manner. Finally, knowledge of normal anatomy, the extent of the defect, and the patient is vital for successful outcomes.

> The esthetic and functional demands of maxillofacial reconstruction have driven the evolution of an array of options. The palatal flap offers a technically simple and predictable option for intraoral reconstruction. Moreover, the palatal island flap is the only available flap that can provide keratinized mucosa for defect reconstruction. Patients usually encounter minimal postoperative morbidity, and should expect a rapid return to a normal diet. Although the palatal flap cannot serve as a panacea for most intraoral reconstruction, it provides the reconstructive surgeon with a great armamentarium.

> The tongue flap is a robust, versatile flap that can be used for reconstruction of oral, pharyngeal, and perioral defects of congenital, traumatic, and ablative origin. The rich blood supply and ease of use make the tongue flap a reliable and predictable reconstructive technique for indicated defects.

> The nasolabial and facial artery musculomucosal (FAMM) flaps are predictable methods to reconstruct perioral and intraoral defects with vascularized tissue. The nasolabial flap can be harvested as an axial or random patterned flap, whereas the FAMM flap is truly an axial patterned flap, with either a superior or an inferior base. Both flaps have been widely used to provide predictable results, with low morbidity. Future studies are needed to further prove their use in compromised patients, including patients with a history of head and neck radiation and neck dissections.

ORAL AND MAXILLOFACIAL SURGERY CLINICS OF NORTH AMERICA

THE CLINICS ARE NOW AVAILABLE ONLINE!
Access your subscription at:
www.theclinics.com

Preface
Local and Regional Flaps of the Head and Neck

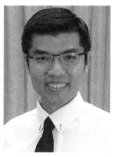 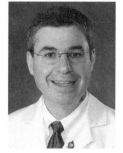

Din Lam, DMD, MD   Robert A. Strauss, DDS, MD
Editors

Over the last decade, few aspects of the specialty of oral and maxillofacial surgery have advanced as much as reconstructive surgery. The advent of microvascular free flaps with or without bone, in particular, has caused a paradigm shift in our ability to reconstruct previously difficult defects due to their size or position. Bony reconstruction of the mandibular midline and long-span osseous defects can now be managed more predictably. Soft tissue free flaps allow for large areas of the head and neck to be reconstructed both functionally and esthetically. However, like most surgical procedures, free flap reconstructions have their downsides. They are technically complex, time-consuming procedures with significant potential for morbidity and failure. In addition, some patients are not candidates for free flaps due to vascular compromise, age, or comorbidities.

Local and regional flaps have long been used for reconstruction in the head and neck. Due to the extensive blood supply in the head and neck, these flaps are generally safe and predictable. Smaller procedures, such as the facial artery myomuscular flap (FAMM flap), platysma flap, tongue flap, paramedian forehead, and nasolabial flaps, can be used when the defect does not call for large tissue mass. In addition, these flaps are relatively easy and quick and are capable of being performed by most oral and maxillofacial surgeons. Larger procedures, such as the pectoralis major and latissimus dorsi flap, can be used as primary reconstructive flaps in patients not suited for free flap reconstruction or as salvage procedures after failure of free flaps.

Having at least some of these procedures in their armamentarium will benefit every surgeon. The cancer reconstructive surgeon will most certainly need the pectoralis major flap sooner or later, but even those surgeons that primarily perform intraoral surgery will gain from having experience with palatal, FAMM, and tongue flaps. During the course of their career, every surgeon experiences that moment when they find themselves facing a soft tissue defect during or after surgery that defies primary closure, by design or unexpectedly. It is both prudent and comforting to have knowledge of some or all of these local and regional flaps when in that situation.

We were very fortunate to have such a distinguished group of authors agree to contribute to this issue of *Oral and Maxillofacial Surgery Clinics of North America*. We are truly grateful for their willingness to participate. In addition, all guest editors of *Oral and Maxillofacial Surgery Clinics of North America* rely on John Vassallo and Yonah Korngold, the resident editors at Elsevier, who

Oral Maxillofacial Surg Clin N Am 26 (2014) xi–xii
http://dx.doi.org/10.1016/j.coms.2014.06.001
1042-3699/14/$ – see front matter © 2014 Published by Elsevier Inc.

oralmaxsurgery.theclinics.com

provide expert advice and guidance. Without them, this issue would not have been possible.

Robert A. Strauss, DDS, MD
Department of Oral and Facial Surgery
Virginia Commonwealth University Medical Center
PO Box 980566
Richmond, VA 23298-0566, USA

Din Lam, DMD, MD
Department of Oral and Facial Surgery
Virginia Commonwealth University Medical Center
PO Box 980566
Richmond, VA 23298-0566, USA

E-mail addresses:
dlam@vcu.edu (D. Lam)
rstrauss@mcvh-vcu.edu (R.A. Strauss)

Basic Flap Design

Todd A. Schultz, DMD[a,b], Kelly Cunningham, MD[a,c,d],
Jonathan S. Bailey, DMD, MD[a,b,c],*

KEYWORDS

- Local flaps • Advancement flaps • Rotation flaps • Transposition flaps • Interpolated flaps

KEY POINTS

- Closely restore the basic functions and properties of the surgical flap and adjacent tissue.
- Draw out the flap; never burn any bridges, consider all options (the reconstructive ladder).
- Replace like with like.
- Use the esthetic units of the face to guide the reconstructive effort.
- Remember the donor site must be closed in an esthetic and functional manner.
- Be knowledgeable of normal anatomy, the extent of the defect, and the patient.

HISTORY

The first documented repair of a complicated nasal defect with a cheek flap occurred in India in 600 BC by Sushruta Samita. These procedures were continued in India, and it was eventually documented in Western medicine in the late 1700s. Tube flaps, delayed flaps, and transfer flaps were used commonly during the 1500s. These techniques were documented by Tagliacozzi. During World War I, Harold Gilies used tube flaps and delayed flaps with a greater emphasis on blood supply during defect reconstruction. These techniques were refined during the 1950s and again in the 1970s, maintaining an emphasis on both cutaneous and vascular blood supply. During the 1950s and 1960s, surgeons utilized flaps with named blood supplies. During the 1970s, flaps with unnamed blood supplies, musculocutaneous flaps, and eventually free tissue transfers were performed. Fasciocutaneous and osteocutaneous flaps began to be used in the 1980s. During the 1990s, perforator flaps based on small vessels arising from larger named vessels traveling through the adjacent muscular tissue were utilized for reconstruction. Although this article is limited to basic flap design, it is useful to understand the evolution of flaps in reconstructive surgery.

PHYSIOLOGIC CHARACTERISTICS OF SKIN

The skin functions and properties include (1) protection/anatomic barrier; (2) thermoregulation; (3) protection against excessive fluid loss/evaporation; (4) storage areas (eg, lipids and water) for synthesis; (5) sensation center (heat cold, touch, vibration, pressure, injury); and (6) formation of an aesthetic zone, enhancing nonverbal communication/expression.

Complicated wounds on the head and neck often require advanced techniques for ideal closure. The nature of the wound determines the approach for proper closure. The location, size, adjacent structures, etiology (eg, trauma, malignancy, or cosmetic defect), expected functional outcome, and medical comorbidities should all be considered when selecting a specific technique.

The goal of proper flap design is to closely restore the skin's functions and properties.

Disclosures: None.
[a] Department of Surgery, University of Illinois Urbana-Champaign College of Medicine, 611 West Park Street, Urbana, IL 61802, USA; [b] Division of Oral and Maxillofacial Surgery, Carle Foundation Hospital, 611 West Park Street, Urbana, IL 61802, USA; [c] Division of Head and Neck Cancer, Carle Foundation Hospital, 611 West Park Street, Urbana, IL 61802, USA; [d] Division of Otolaryngology, Carle Foundation Hospital, 611 West Park Street, Urbana, IL 61802, USA
* Corresponding author. Division of Oral and Maxillofacial Surgery, Carle Foundation Hospital, 611 West Park Street, Urbana, IL 61802.
E-mail address: jonathan.bailey@carle.com

Oral Maxillofacial Surg Clin N Am 26 (2014) 277–303
http://dx.doi.org/10.1016/j.coms.2014.05.001
1042-3699/14/$ – see front matter © 2014 Elsevier Inc. All rights reserved.

Obviously, an understanding of proper wound closure, wound healing, relaxed skin tension lines, and the facial esthetic zones is essential in this task. Realistic patient expectations are essential to enhance overall patient satisfaction.

PREOPERATIVE CONSIDERATIONS

Preoperative considerations should include: (1) evaluation of smoking history, atherosclerosis, peripheral vascular disease, steroid use, diabetes, and previous surgeries; (2) extent of traumatic injury; (3) patient age and skin condition; and (4) defect location.

The ability of the body to heal and adequately perfuse the adjacent tissue and flap is of paramount importance. A patient who presents with deficits in tissue perfusion or in the ability to heal would lead the surgeon toward a less complicated closure of the defect based on the reconstructive ladder (**Fig. 1**). Therefore, an extensive evaluation of smoking history, atherosclerosis, peripheral vascular disease, steroid use, diabetes, and previous surgeries must be elicited preoperatively. Additionally, evaluation of traumatic injuries must evaluate the size and extent of the wound and

gauge the underlying defect. Defects with exposed bone or compromised arterial or venous systems will also affect the surgeon's closure design. These types of defects may result in compromises in esthetic or functional outcome during defect closure. These circumstances may require advanced reconstructive techniques.

Increased patient age and accumulated skin damage decrease skin elasticity and moisture content. Even though the quality of skin may decrease with age, wrinkles often conceal scars effectively. Usually wrinkles are found within the relaxed skin tension lines or RSTLs (**Fig. 2**). RSTLs are determined by the orientation of collagen fibers. These lines are perpendicular to the lines of maximal extensibility. Knowledge of these lines is essential for cosmetic and functional wound closure.

Wound location often increases the complexity of wound closure. The areas that usually cause the greatest concern are the nasal tip/alar complex, eyelids, vermilion border, and the external ear (**Box 1**). Each of these areas is considered to be within specific esthetic zones of the face (**Fig. 3**). Typically, the skin in each esthetic zone is considered to have similar qualities of texture, pigmentation, elasticity, and thickness. Ideally, local skin with similar qualities is used to reconstruct facial defects. Flap designs that utilize

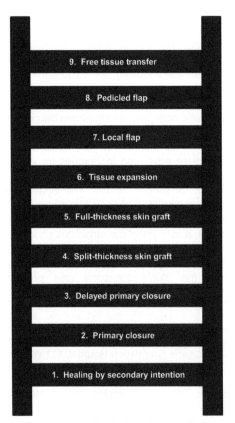

Fig. 1. The reconstructive ladder. Complexity increases as the surgeon goes up the ladder.

9. Free tissue transfer

8. Pedicled flap

7. Local flap

6. Tissue expansion

5. Full-thickness skin graft

4. Split-thickness skin graft

3. Delayed primary closure

2. Primary closure

1. Healing by secondary intention

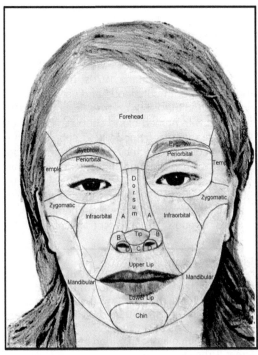

Fig. 2. Esthetic zones for the face. (A) Lateral nasal wall. (B) Nasal ala. (C) Columella. (D) Anterior nares soft tissue.

similar skin types and conceal scars in the esthetic unit boundaries are ideal. However, in these difficult areas, special consideration must be given to the reconstructive decision-making process.[1–5]

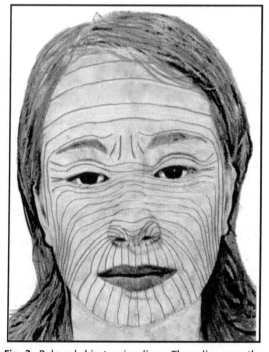

Fig. 3. Relaxed skin tension lines. These lines are the result of adjacent collagen fibers and run perpendicular to the lines of maximum extensibility.

Preoperative knowledge and intraoperative execution of proper tissue handling are also vital to an optimal outcome. Skin margins should be handled below the level of the epidermis with skin hooks or fine-toothed forceps to avoid trauma. The flap's vascular supply should not be compromised by technique or design. Sharp angles or kinking should be avoided at the base of any planned flap. Tension-free closure is required for optimizing wound healing and maintaining vascularity. Adequate mobilization of the flap and adjacent tissue can minimize tension. Additionally, the surgeon must plan to provide thorough surgical site hemostasis to avoid hematoma and resultant necrosis. Meticulous preoperative planning and intraoperative execution are required to obtain optimal postoperative results.

FLAP NOMENCLATURE

The description of a wound starts with the primary defect. The primary defect is produced after the removal of a neoplastic lesion or the result of trauma. The primary defect is often revised in preparation of a specific flap design. A secondary defect is the wound that is left after adjacent tissue is transferred to close the primary defect. Movement of a flap toward the defect in an effort to close the primary defect is a description of primary movement. Mobilization of tissue adjacent to the primary defect and advancement toward the center of the defect describe secondary movement.

Classification of flaps may be defined by the configuration, tissue layers, blood supply, region, and method of transfer. Tissue configuration describes the geometric shape of the flap. These flaps include rhomboid, bilobed, z-plasty, v-y, rotation, and others. Flaps can also be classified by their tissue content. These flaps include: cutaneous (skin and subcutaneous tissue), myocutaneous (composite of skin, muscle, and blood supply), and fasciocutanous (deep muscle fascia, skin, regional artery perforators). Arterial supply can be used to classify a cutaneous flap as a random pattern, axial pattern, or pedicle flap (**Fig. 4**). The most common type is the random pattern, which uses the dermal and subdermal plexus as its blood supply. Dominant vessels oriented in a superficial axial position are used to supply blood in an axial pattern flap. Pedicle flaps often use named arteries (through muscular perforators). If the flap is harvested from a distant site, and the vascular supply is reestablished at the defect site, it is defined as a free tissue transfer.

Classification can also be based on the relative location of the donor site. Local flaps are considered adjacent to the primary defect. Regional

A

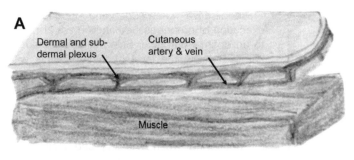

Dermal and sub-
dermal plexus

Cutaneous
artery & vein

Muscle

B

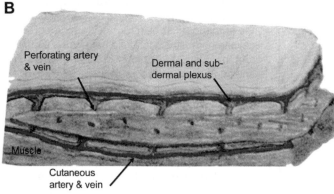

Perforating artery
& vein

Dermal and sub-
dermal plexus

Muscle

Cutaneous
artery & vein

Fig. 4. (*A*) Axial pattern flap. (*B*) Random pattern flap.

flap donor sites are located on different areas of the same body part. If different body parts are used as the donor site, the flap is termed a distant flap.

Description of the flap movement is the most common method of classifying reconstructive techniques. Advancement flaps, rotation flaps, transposition flaps, interposition flaps, and interpolated flaps are common techniques. Advancement flaps use mobilized tissue in a direction toward the primary defect. Rotation flaps pivot mobilized tissue around a point toward the primary defect. Transposition flaps are mobilized tissues that traverse adjacent tissue by rotation and/or advancement in an effort to close the primary defect. When the adjacent tissue is also mobilized to close a defect by secondary movement, the flap is classified as an interposition flap. Interpolated flaps are mobilized tissues that traverse over or beneath an otherwise noncompromised skin bridge in the form of a pedicle to close the primary defect. The pedicle consists of skin (possibly subcutaneous fat and muscle) and/or an individual artery and vein used, with adjacent tissue, to maintain vascularity of the flap. At least 1 additional procedure is required to divide a pedicle. Finally, microvascular free tissue transfer utilizes tissue transferred from a different part of the body and requires a microvascular anastomosis with an adjacent vascular supply to provide tissue to close the primary defect.

LOCAL FLAPS
Advancement Flaps

Advancement flaps have a linear configuration. They are mobilized and usually travel in a single vector toward the defect. These flaps can approach the defect from one or more sides of the defect for closure. Advancement flaps work best in areas of the head and neck with greater skin elasticity.[6] When the resultant scar can be hidden within natural skin creases, this flap design is preferred. Most of the wound tension is oriented within the advancement vector (on the distal flap margin). Therefore, tension is limited in a vector parallel to the flap advancement. This condition is most advantageous when distortion must be limited adjacent to the primary defect. Advancement flaps include: unipedicle or unilateral advancement flaps, bilateral unipedicle advancement flaps, bipedicle advancement flaps, y-v advancement flaps, v-y advancement flaps, and island advancement flaps.

In designing a unipedicle or unilateral advancement flap, the width is based on the width of the primary defect (**Figs. 5–13**). Two incisions are developed parallel in nature to produce the length of the flap. The total length of the flap should be 1.5 to 3 times the defect width.[7–9] Complete undermining from the distal to the proximal aspect of the flap is required. Undermining the defect margins is recommended. Removal of standing cutaneous deformities (dog-ears) with z-plasty, inverse triangular

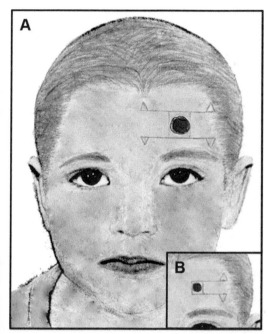

Fig. 5. (*A*) Design for a bilateral unipedicle advancement flap. (*B*) Design for a unipedicle advancement flap.

skin excisions, or Burow triangles near the corners of the flap base is usually required. The standing cutaneous deformities can be corrected at any point along the length of the initial parallel incisions.

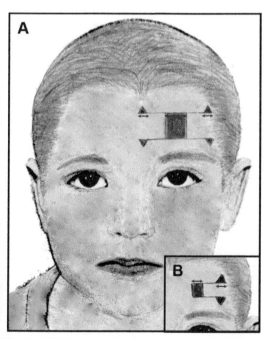

Fig. 6. (*A*) Bilateral unipedicle advancement flap. (*B*) Unipedicle advancement flap. Note, the Burow triangle length (sum) should equal the defect length. Flap length is 1.5× to 3× the primary defect length.

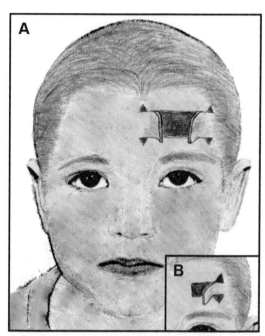

Fig. 7. (*A*) Bilateral unipedicle advancement flap (undermining the flap). (*B*) Unipedicle advancement flap (undermining the flap).

This flap does not create a secondary defect. Repair of the primary defect involves both primary and secondary tissue movement. Unipedicle advancement flaps are often used on the forehead (especially the

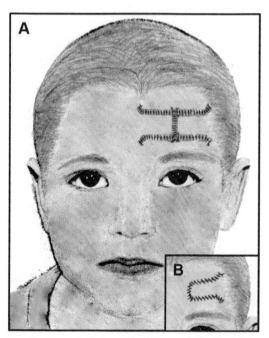

Fig. 8. (*A*) Bilateral unipedicle advancement flap (wound sutured). (*B*) Unipedicle advancement flap (wound sutured).

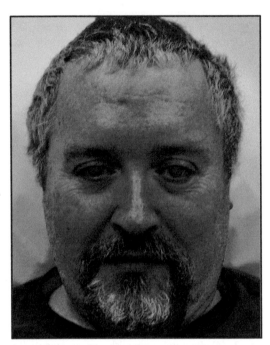

Fig. 9. 49-year-old man with a shave biopsy-proven basal cell carcinoma on the right side of his forehead.

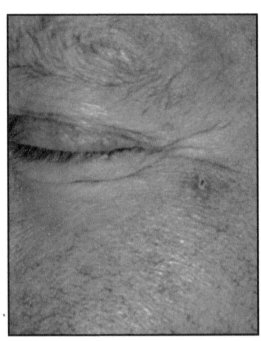

Fig. 11. 76-year-old man with a shave biopsy-proven basal cell carcinoma on the left lateral periorbital area.

hair line and eyebrow areas), the upper and lower eyelids, the medial cheek, the vermilion, within the oral cavity, and the helical rim.

Bilateral unipedicle advancement flaps approach the defect from opposite sides to close

the wound (see **Figs. 5–8**). The combination of the 2 flaps is used to close the primary defect. In general, the same principles are used that were previously discussed with unipedicle flap design.

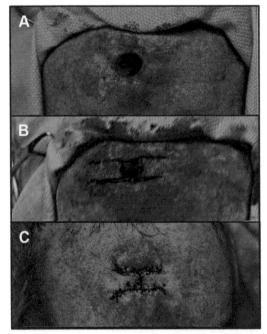

Fig. 10. (A) Development of the primary defect. (B) Development of H-plasty flaps. (C) Sutured H-plasty.

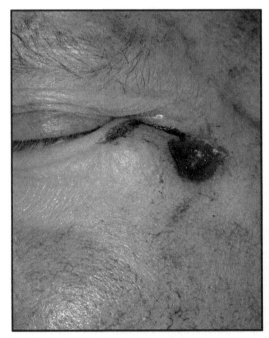

Fig. 12. Creation of the primary defect and design of unipedicle advancement flap (within skin crease of the lower eyelid).

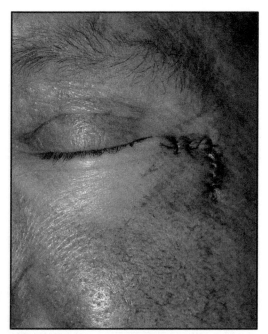

Fig. 13. Closure of the unipedicle advancement flap (within skin crease of the lower eyelid).

However, the resultant repair is H- or T-shaped. The procedures are usually referred to as H-plasty (see **Figs. 5–8**) or T-plasty (**Figs. 14–16**). These flaps are used in similar locations as unipedicle advancement flaps.

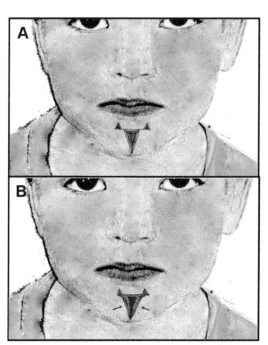

Fig. 15. (*A*) Note, the Burrow's triangle length (sum) should equal the defect width. (*B*) The lateral edges will be advanced medially in the A-T flap (as noted with the *arrows*).

Bipedicle advancement flaps repairs are rarely utilized on the head and neck. This flap does have indications for closure of scalp wounds and full-thickness defects involving the nasal tip or

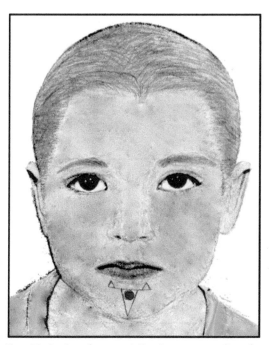

Fig. 14. Design for an A-T advancement flap for closure of a mental crease defect.

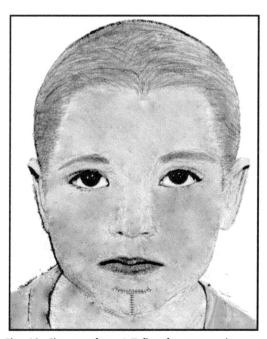

Fig. 16. Closure of an A-T flap for a mental crease defect.

ala (with a vertical height of <1 cm). The design of this flap is oriented adjacent to the defect. The flap is advanced into the primary defect at a right angle. This technique requires the use of a split-thickness skin graft to cover the resultant second-ary defect.

v-y advancement flaps use a mobilized v-shaped flap that pushes away from the primary defect. The resultant area is a chevron-shaped defect. The adjacent margins of the resultant defect are also mobilized and then used to close the defect. The resultant y-shaped repaired defect represents a nearly tension-free closure (**Figs. 17–19**). Attempts to place the limbs of the y-shaped repaired inci-sions within natural skin creases add to the esthetic quality of the flap. This flap design is used on de-fects of the lateral nasal ala. Furthermore, this flap can be used to repair scars that distort the hairline, vermilion border, or eyelids. The scar causing the defect should be incorporated into the superior aspect of the original v-shaped flap. Therefore, this area will move superiorly to correct the defect.

y-v advancement flaps have the opposite move-ment of the adjacent mobilized tissue seen in the v-y advancement flap. The mobilized tissue within the original y-shaped area is advanced into the resultant primary defect and the apex of the v-shaped structure. The lateral mobilized tissue

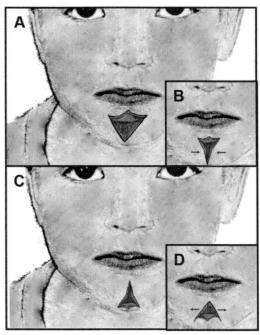

Fig. 18. (*A–D*) Development of the revised primary defect. (*B*) The lateral edges will be advanced medially and the superior edge superiorly in the v-y flap (as noted with the *arrows*). (*D*) The lateral edges will be advanced laterally and the superior edge inferiorly in the y-v flap (as noted with the *arrows*).

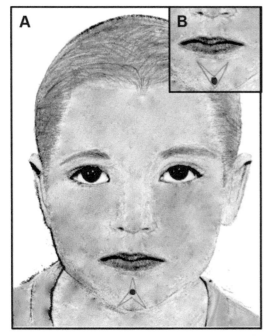

Fig. 17. (*A*) Design for a y-v advancement flap for closure of a mental crease defect. (*B*) Design for a v-y advancement flap for closure of a chin defect.

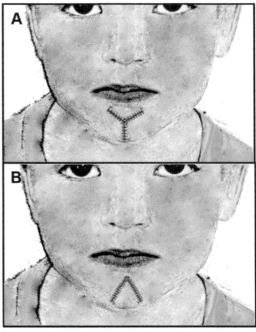

Fig. 19. (*A*) Closure of a y-v advancement flap for closure of a mental crease defect. (*B*) Closure a v-y advancement flap for closure of a chin defect.

is pushed outward (see **Figs. 17–19**). Although use of this flap design is more limited, it can be used to correct a medially scarred oral commissure.

Island flaps can be based on a hinge movement, a linear advancement movement, or a combination of the two. Island flaps used on the head and neck usually follow a linear advancement pattern. Island flaps are designed by freeing an area of cutaneous tissue on all borders (**Figs. 20–28**). The island maintains its dermal and subcutaneous attachments along with a vascular supply. The cutaneous island is carefully undermined to the extent required to bring it into the primary defect site without compromising the blood supply. The cutaneous island can be shaped like a triangle, square, rectangle, or circle. v-y shaped island flaps and island flaps based on hinge movement have decreased wound closure tension. Usually, the most tension is found perpendicular to a leading margin of the island flap. The repaired defect will have a sutured area around the cutaneous island along with a sutured linear or curvilinear tail. These flaps are often used in defects found along the nasal–labial fold, nasal ala, cheek, and periorbital area.

Rotation Flaps

In contrast to advancement flaps, rotation flaps have a curvilinear configuration and rotate around a central point. The defect is located within the arc of rotation. These flaps can be useful in areas of

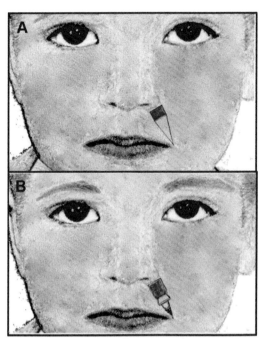

Fig. 21. (*A*) Creation of the revised primary defect. Incision on the periphery of the island. (*B*) Undermining the leading and trailing edges to create the island flap.

decreased skin elasticity. It is often more difficult to hide these flaps within existing skin creases. In designing the flap, after the final margins of the primary defect are established, the defect is revised

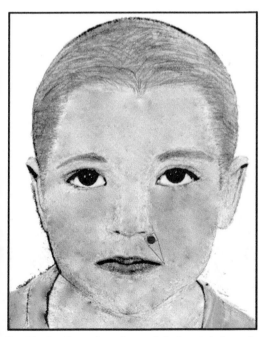

Fig. 20. Creation of a primary defect and design of a v-y island flap to close a left nasal–labial crease defect.

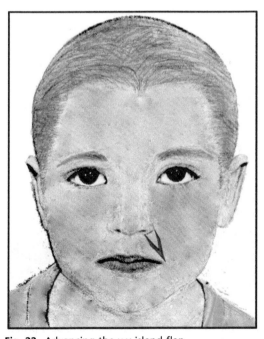

Fig. 22. Advancing the v-y island flap.

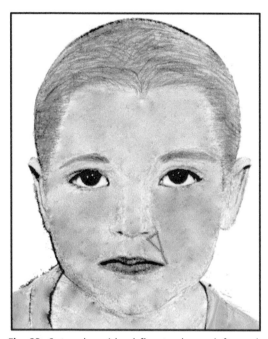

Fig. 23. Sutured v-y island flap to close a left nasal–labial crease defect.

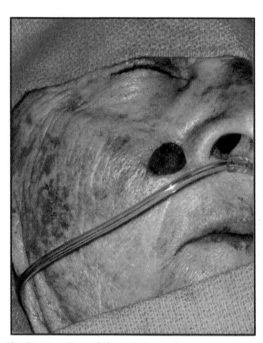

Fig. 25. Creation of the primary defect.

into an arc. The curved segment of the arc is continuous with a curvilinear incision. In designing a rotation flap, it is important to remember rotation of the flap decreases the effective length of the flap. For example, flap rotation of 90° reduces the flap length by 15%; rotation of 45° reduces the length by 5%.[10] A releasing incision on the opposite end of the curvilinear incision can be

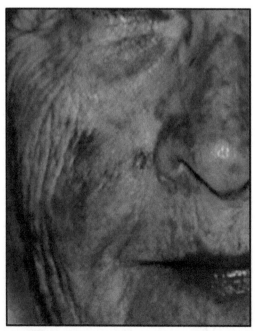

Fig. 24. 78-year-old woman with a biopsy-proven basal cell carcinoma on the right nasal–labial crease.

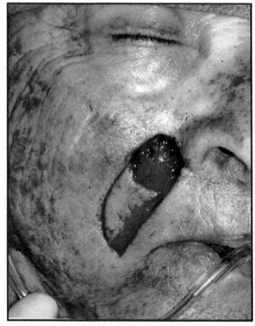

Fig. 26. Creation of the island flap within the nasal–labial crease.

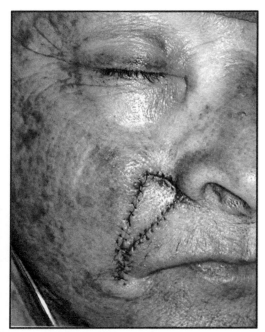

Fig. 27. Closure of the v-y island flap of the right nasal–labial crease.

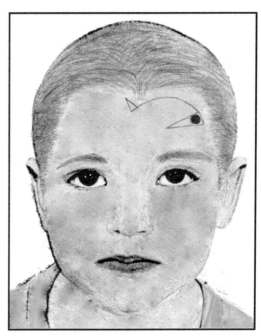

Fig. 29. Creation of a primary defect and design of a rotation flap to close a left lateral forehead defect.

used to gain additional length (**Figs. 29–34**). If this releasing incision is made, it is imperative that the vascular supply to the flap is not compromised. Undermining from the distal to the proximal aspect

of the flap is required. Undermining the adjacent flap and defect tissue is recommended. Removal of standing cutaneous deformities with z-plasty, inverse triangular skin excisions, or Burow

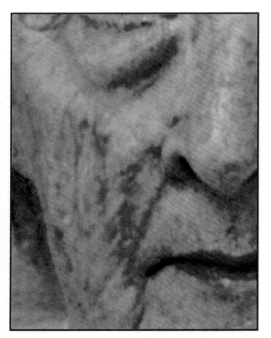

Fig. 28. Postoperative view of v-y island flap on right nasal–labial crease at 2 weeks.

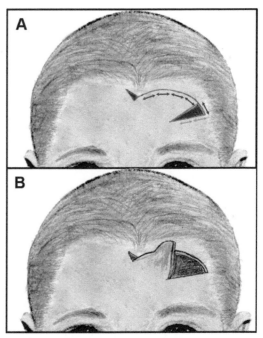

Fig. 30. (*A*) The curvilinear distance of the rotation flap should be 4× the defect width (*red double arrows*). The arc length should be at least 2× the width (*yellow double arrows*). (*B*) Undermined flap edges.

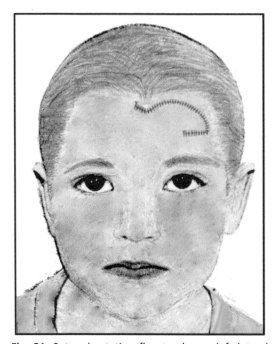

Fig. 31. Sutured rotation flap to close a left lateral forehead defect.

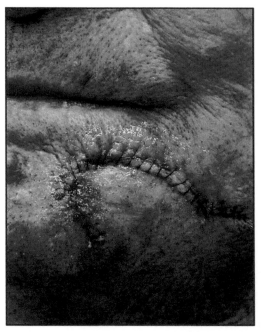

Fig. 33. Rotation flap design for closure of a primary defect.

triangles may be required. The standing cutaneous deformities can be corrected at any point along the length of the curvilinear incision. However, avoidance of these deformities may be the best option.

Usually, designing a flap with a curvilinear distance of 4 times the width of the revised defect arc will limit standing cutaneous deformities within the curvilinear aspect of the rotation flap. Additionally,

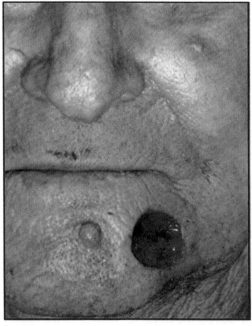

Fig. 32. 76-year-old man with shave biopsy-proven basal cell carcinoma of the left lateral chin area. Primary defect.

Fig. 34. Sutured closure of a rotation flap (left lateral chin).

standing cutaneous deformities can be limited at the base of the rotation flap by designing the revised arc (modification of the primary defect) with a height 2 times the maximum width.[6] If a standing cutaneous deformity is noted at the base, and there is concern about the vascular supply of the flap, the deformity should be left in place and a second-stage revision procedure planned. These flaps are commonly used on the nasal dorsum and the scalp.[2,11] On the scalp, the rotation flap can be combined with 1 or 2 additional rotation flaps for closure. This situation is usually referred to as a double-rotation (o-z) flap or a triple rotation flap (**Figs. 35–40**).

Transposition Flaps

Transposition flaps are considered to be one of the most common methods for transferring tissue on the head and neck. Traditionally, these flaps are rotated over adjacent tissue and advanced to close a defect. Similar to a rotation flap, it is important to remember rotation of the flap decreases the effective length of the flap. The same estimates for reduction in elective length apply. Examples of this flap include bilobed transposition flaps (double transposition flap) and rhomboid transposition flaps (Linberg flaps). In general, the length of the flap should not exceed 3 times the width. The patient's ability to adequately perfuse the tissue and the tissue quality must be considered if this

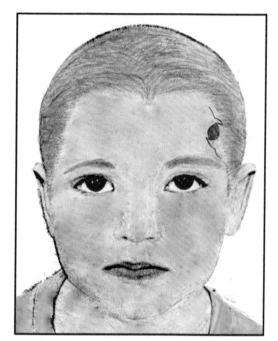

Fig. 36. Undermined flap edges on a double rotation flap.

guideline is exceeded. Usually, the flap is designed so that the base of the flap is the only part continuous with the primary (or revised) defect. The greatest amount of tension within the secondary defect closure site is near the adjacent point of rotation

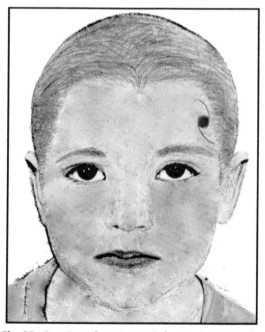

Fig. 35. Creation of a primary defect and design of a double rotation flap (o-z) to close a left lateral forehead defect.

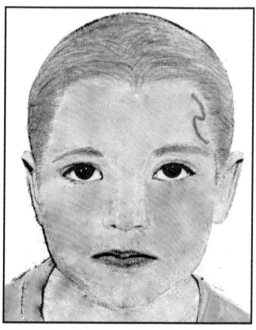

Fig. 37. Sutured double rotation flap to close a left lateral forehead defect.

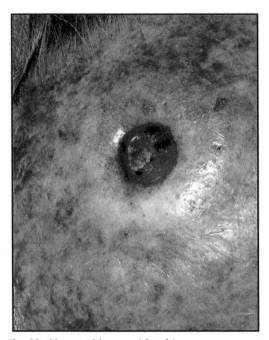

Fig. 38. 92-year-old man with a biopsy-proven squamous cell carcinoma on the left posterior scalp (balding male). Primary defect.

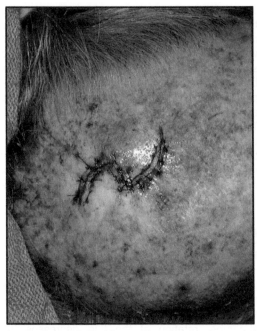

Fig. 40. Sutured double rotation flap to close a left posterior scalp defect.

at the base of the flap. Areas of increased skin elasticity are more conducive to this type of flap. Due to the shape of this flap, it is usually difficult to hide the flap closure entirely within natural skin creases.

Bilobed transposition flaps are designed with a single base and 2 lobe transposition flaps attached (**Figs. 41–50**). The classic bilobed flap has 2 separate pivot points. The donor sites are

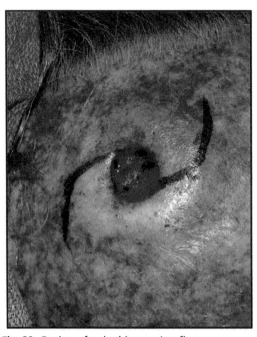

Fig. 39. Design of a double rotation flap.

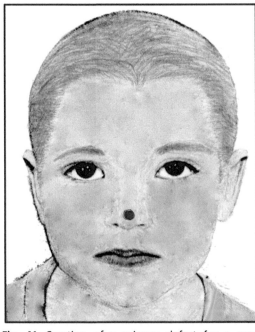

Fig. 41. Creation of a primary defect for a nasal defect.

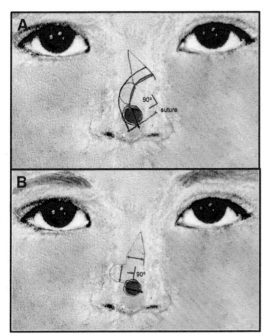

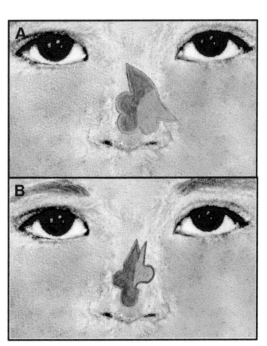

Fig. 42. (*A*) Design of a bilobed transposition flap (45° between the lobes, the width of the lobes is equal). A suture can be used to create an arc at the edge and middle of the lobes). (*B*) Classic design of a bilobed transposition flap (90° between the lobes; the width of the lobes is equal).

Fig. 44. (*A, B*) Undermined biloped flaps.

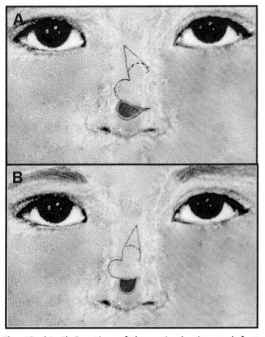

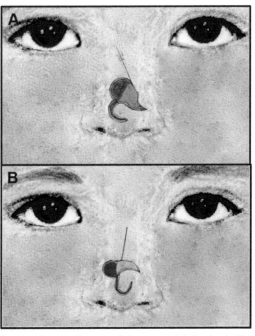

Fig. 43. (*A, B*) Creation of the revised primary defect.

Fig. 45. (*A, B*) Closure of the second lobe (*arc*). The second donor lobe (*arc*) is maintained.

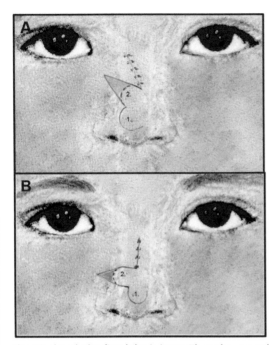

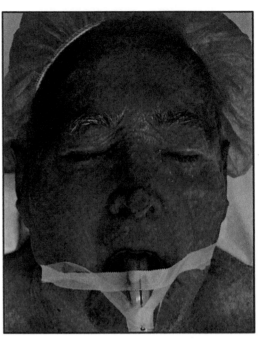

Fig. 46. (*A, B*) The first lobe is inset. Then the second arc is trimmed to match the secondary defect before it is inset.

Fig. 48. 60-year-old man with biopsy-proven basal cell carcinoma on the nasal tip.

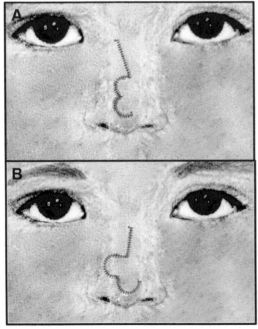

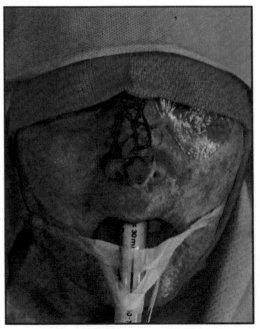

Fig. 47. (*A, B*) Sutured closure of the bilobed transposition flaps.

Fig. 49. Design of a bilobed transposition flap and primary defect.

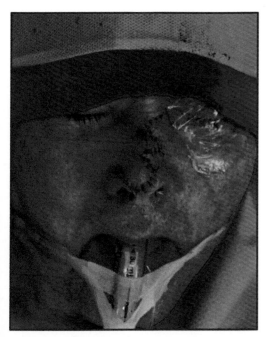

Fig. 50. Sutured bilobed transposition flap for closure of a nasal tip defect.

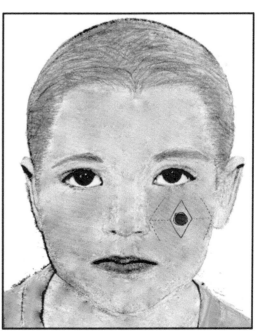

Fig. 51. Creation of a primary defect and design of a rhomboid transposition flap to close a left cheek defect. Note, the rhomboid can be rotated in all directions to create the optimal design. Once the primary defect is revised (**Fig. 53**A), there are 4 possible flap donor sites.

90° from the original defect and each other. The width of the first lobed donor site and the second triangular donor site should be equal to the original defect width. The 2 lobes are mobilized and placed within the primary and secondary defects. An alternative method uses a single pivot point for both lobes. The lobes are 45° apart. The width of the 2 lobes is still established by the primary defect. After the 2 lobes are mobilized, the defect created by the second lobe (triangle) is closed. Next, the triangle is trimmed to fit the secondary defect. Finally, the primary defect is modified to a lobe (arc) shape, and the first donor lobe is inset. This flap is frequently used on defects less than or equal to 1.5 cm on the nasal tip, nasal dorsum, and nasal ala.[6] However, this flap can be used for cheek and forehead defects also. Caution should be taken when using these flaps, as a narrow pedicle can cause congestion. The circular nature of the flap and/or the thickness of the flap can decrease the esthetic result.

Rhomboid transposition flaps are initiated by transforming the primary defect into a parallelogram (**Figs. 51–59**). The internal angles of the defect should measure 60° (on opposite sides) and 120° (on opposite sides). This defect has

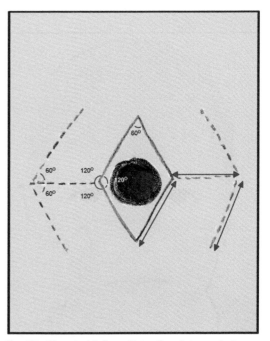

Fig. 52. Rhomboid flap. Note the distance between the double arrows should be equal on each line segment. The flap should be constructed approximately with 120° and 60° angles.

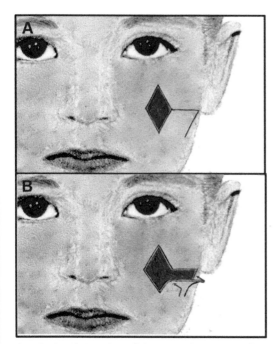

Fig. 53. (A, B) Creation of the revised primary defect. The flap with an ideal donor site is chosen and under-mined (movement indicated by *arrows*).

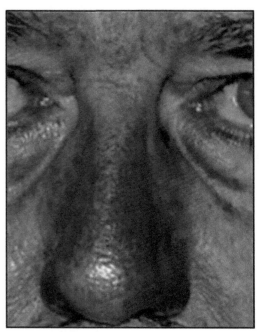

Fig. 55. 60-year old man with a biopsy-proven basal cell carcinoma on the left superior lateral nasal wall.

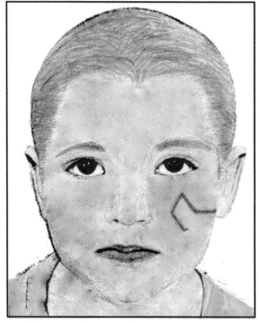

Fig. 54. Sutured closure of a rhomboid transposition flap to close a left cheek defect.

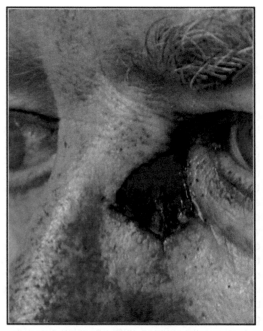

Fig. 56. Primary defect after frozen sections.

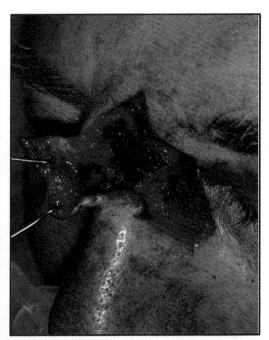

Fig. 57. Creation of the revised primary defect. The flap with an ideal donor site is chosen and undermined.

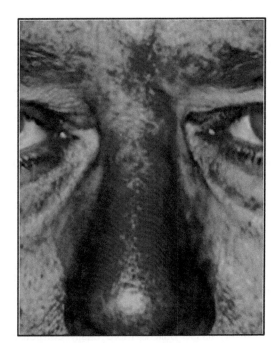

Fig. 59. One month postoperatively.

4 possible donor sites (2 on each 120° corner). An incision is made at the 120° corner. This incision should measure 120° from the adjacent defect border. The length of the incision is variable. The more closely the distance mirrors the length of the defect between the corners of the parallelogram, the less tension experienced at the revised primary defect closure site. The compromise is a larger secondary defect. A second incision is made at approximately 30° to 60° from the previously mentioned incision.[6,12] Again, the tradeoff is potentially greater tension adjacent to the revised primary defect or a larger secondary defect and increased tension at the secondary defect closure site. The length of the incision should closely mirror the length of the defect between the corners of the parallelogram. The flap is then undermined and inserted in the revised primary defect site. Undermining the adjacent tissue has minimal effect of skin tension. These flaps are often used on the cheek and periauricular area, and the anterior/lateral neck.

With both rhomboid transposition flaps and bilobed transposition flaps, if a standing cutaneous deformity is noted, and there is concern about the vascular supply of the flap, the deformity should be left in place and a second stage revision procedure planned. Otherwise, standing cutaneous deformities can be treated as mentioned with previous flaps. It may be difficult to camouflage the closure within natural skin creases. An additional downside to using these flaps is the large amount of discarded tissue.

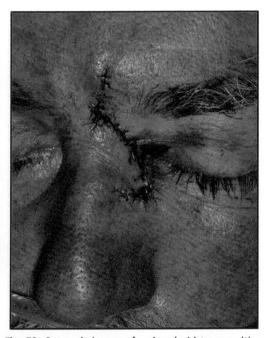

Fig. 58. Sutured closure of a rhomboid transposition flap to close a left lateral nasal area.

Interpolated Flaps

Interpolated flaps use rotational and linear movement to repair a primary defect. The flap does not have a base next to the defect. The flap traverses above or below adjacent tissue, while connected to the base with a pedicle, to close the primary defect. If the pedicle travels superficial to adjacent cutaneous tissue, at least 1 additional procedure is required to remove the pedicle. If this technique is used, the surgeon must be careful to prevent as much tension as possible at the base to limit flap congestion. Additionally, if the surgeon decides to place the pedicle beneath the adjacent tissue (modified island flap), adequate space must be prepared in the adjacent subcutaneous tissue to accommodate the pedicle. The surgeon must be concerned about compression from the adjacent tissue and the superficial layers of the skin causing congestion. Tissue bulk can be a concern if the pedicle is superficial or tunneled. However, tissue bulk is more easily corrected with the superficial approach. The superficial approach also allows the vascular integrity of the flap to be more easily monitored. The most

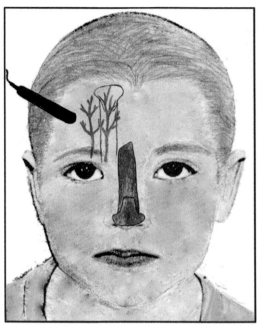

Fig. 61. A template is used to design the interpolated paramedian forehead flap. The supertrochlear and superorbital arteries can be mapped with a Doppler ultrasound. The design is drawn on the forehead.

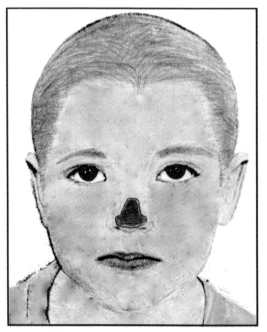

Fig. 60. Creation of a primary defect for a large nasal defect.

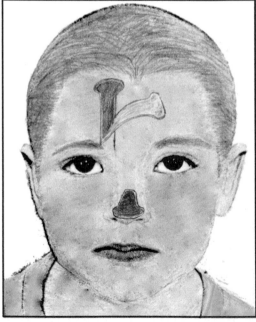

Fig. 62. The flap is undermined while maintaining vascularity.

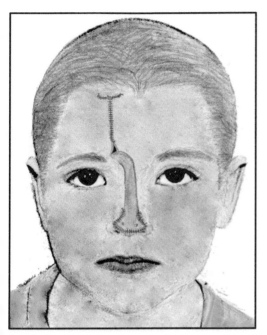

Fig. 63. The interpolated paramedian forehead flap is inset over the nasal defect. If possible, the forehead is primarily closed. Note, the vascularity of the flap must be maintained (use caution when suturing near the base, frequently check the flap with Doppler ultrasound).

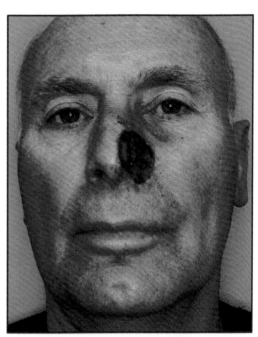

Fig. 65. Front view of a primary defect of a biopsy-proven basal cell carcinoma on the left lateral nasal border, tip, and ala of a 66 year old man.

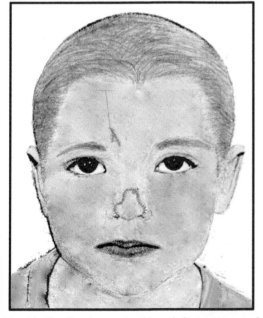

Fig. 64. The flap is usually thinned during a second operative procedure at approximately 3 weeks. During the final procedure (up to 3 weeks after the revision), the base of the pedicle is trimmed and inset to restore proper eyebrow esthetics. The superior edge of the nasal donor tissue is inset and sutured.

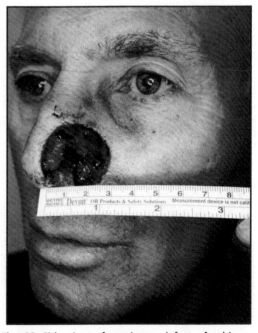

Fig. 66. Side view of a primary defect of a biopsy-proven basal cell carcinoma on the left lateral nasal border, tip, and ala of a 66-year-old man.

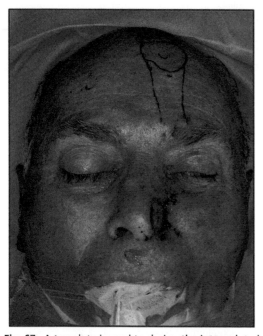

Fig. 67. A template is used to design the interpolated paramedian forehead flap. The supertrochlear and superorbital arteries were mapped with Doppler ultrasound. The design was drawn on the forehead.

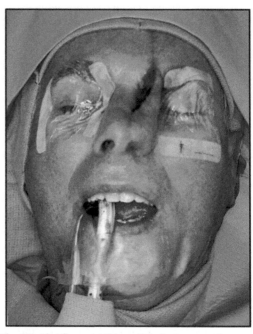

Fig. 68. The flap was thinned during a second operative procedure at approximately 3 weeks.

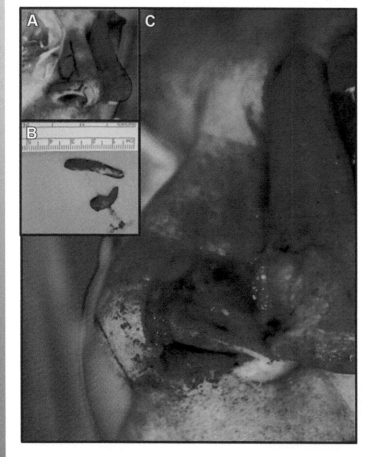

Fig. 69. (*A–C*) Cartilage from the ear was used to provide support by functionally replacing the nasal cartilage.

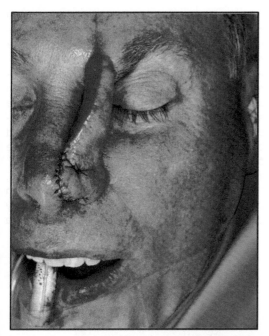

Fig. 70. The interpolated paramedian forehead flap was sutured after the cartilage graft was placed and the flap thinned.

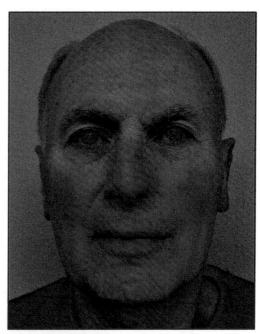

Fig. 72. One year postoperatively (interpolated paramedian forehead flap).

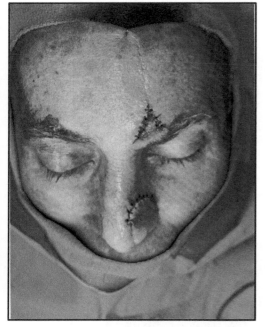

Fig. 71. During the final procedure the base of the pedicle is trimmed and inset to restore proper eyebrow esthetics. The superior edge of the nasal donor tissue is inset and sutured.

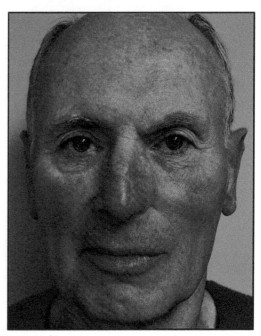

Fig. 73. 2$\frac{1}{2}$ years postoperatively (interpolated paramedian forehead flap).

common types of interpolated flaps utilized in the head and neck region are the paramedian forehead flap (for large defects of the nasal tip and nasal dorsum defects) and melolabial interpolated flap (for large defects of the nasal ala and surrounding tissue). While the paramedian forehead flap crosses the natural creases of the forehead in a perpendicular manner, the secondary defect repair tends to heal well. Additionally, the melolabial interpolated flap has an exceptional esthetic result due to the fact that it is centered on the nasolabial crease. The disadvantages of these flaps are the need for multiple procedures and the interim esthetic compromise the patient must endure.

Paramedian forehead flaps utilize the axial blood supply provided by the supratrochlear artery and vein (the supraorbital artery and vein or random pattern variants can be used if the supratrochlear vascularity has been previously compromised). While designing this flap, the surgeon should trace the primary defect and transfer a slightly larger image (on sterile paper) on the superior portion of the forehead. The pedicle should be drawn after conformation of the course of the supratrochlear artery with Doppler ultrasound. The pedicle width should be 1 to 1.5 cm. Then, the final location of the sterile paper can be drawn on the skin after it is adjusted to the previously drawn pedicle. The flap is then harvested in a

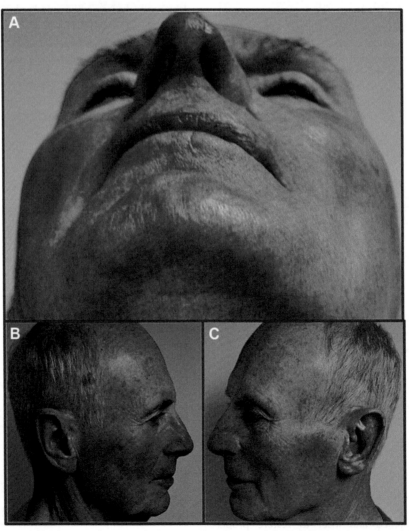

Fig. 74. 2½ years postoperatively (interpolated paramedian forehead flap). (*A*) Worms-eye view. (*B*) Right lateral view. (*C*) Left lateral view.

subgaleal or subcutaneous plane. The skin paddle can be thinned at this point or during a subsequent procedure (if there are concerns about maintaining vascularity). The pedicle can be divided after approximately 3 weeks. To enhance eyebrow symmetry, the base of the pedicle should be inset back into the glabellar area (**Figs. 60–74**).

Melolabial interpolated flaps are used to close defects on the lower third of the lateral nose (ala area). The flap can be based on the angular artery, infraorbital artery, or infratrochlear artery. The flap can be based on random blood supply. Similar to the paramedian forehead flap, the design is drawn out, and the flap is harvested. The skin paddle can be thinned at this point or during a subsequent procedure (if there are concerns about maintaining vascularity). The pedicle can be divided after approximately 3 weeks (if random blood supply is used, 3 weeks is the minimum amount of time before division is recommended).

Interpolated flaps also include ear flaps (pedicle helix reconstruction), lip-switch flaps (Abbe), and tongue flaps. Ear flaps can be based on axial pattern, random pattern, or named vascular supply depending on the size of the defect and the pedicle length (**Figs. 75–78**). The pedicle is divided after 3 weeks. Lip-switch flaps are used to move tissue from the upper or lower lip to a defect located on the opposite lip. This flap can be used to reconstruct one-fourth of the upper lip and one-third of the lower lip. The vascular supply is usually based on the labial artery.[13–15] The pedicle is divided after 2 to 3 weeks. Similarly, the tongue flap is an interpolated flap that can be used to repair intraoral defects. The lingual artery, along with axial and collateral circulation, make this flap a great donor source for restoring intraoral defect or oral antral fistulas. This procedure has minimal impingement of mastication, speech, or deglutition.[16] The biggest concern when using these procedures is the heavy reliance on patient compliance.

COMPLICATIONS

Complications can be divided into early and late in nature. Early complications usually occur in the time frame right after the procedure to as long as the first couple months after the procedure. Late complications usually take longer to mature.

Early complications most commonly involve seroma formation, wound dehiscence, hematoma, and infection.[17] Although most of these complications can be limited with proper technique and design, a limited number will require early

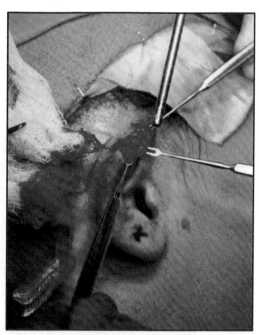

Fig. 75. Primary defect after a dog bite on the right helix and antihelix of an 8-year-old girl.

intervention. Flap necrosis is a more serious complication and usually arises due to errors in design that cause limited blood flow through the flap. This situation can be caused by excessive

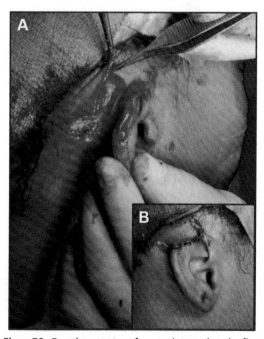

Fig. 76. Development of an interpolated flap advanced onto the right helix and antihelix (*A*) and sutured in place (*B*).

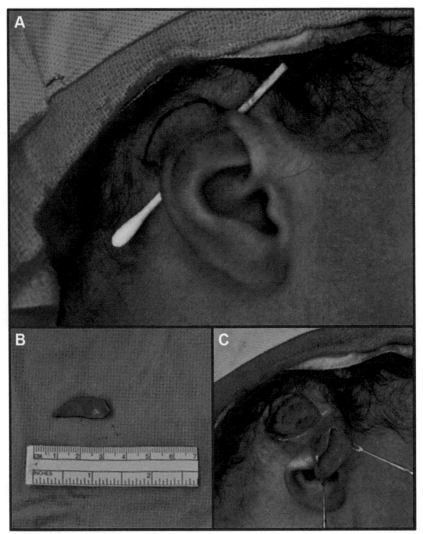

Fig. 77. (*A*) Pedicle on the right helix and antihelix after 3 weeks. (*B*) Cartilage graft from right conchal bowl. (*C*) Division of the pedicle.

tension, interruption in normal blood flow (trauma, patient factors, surgical damage), and narrow and/or long flap design. Areas of less esthetic or functional concern can heal by secondary intention and can be revised at a later date. Areas on the opposite end of the spectrum, such as eyelids, should be revised as soon as possible.

Late complications usually involve scars, pincushioning deformity, hypertrophic scars, and keloid formation.[17] Scar formation can be limited by proper flap design, knowledge of RSTLs, the zones of facial esthetics, proper tissue handling, and appropriate postoperative care. Evaluation of the patient's history of scar formation (including hypertrophic scars and keloid formation) is extremely important. Options for treatment of hypertrophic scars (and scars in general) are excision, z-plasty, and w-plasty. Scars and pincushioning deformities can also revised by defatting the flap or adjacent tissue. These treatment techniques should not be performed until the wound matures. Keloids (if known to form from patient history or recognized early) can be treated with pressure, massage, and steroid injections. Some authors also advocate use of topical silicone. Once the keloid forms, excision with steroid injections within the lesion can be utilized. Patients should be advised that the keloid could increase in size, and this communication should be documented.

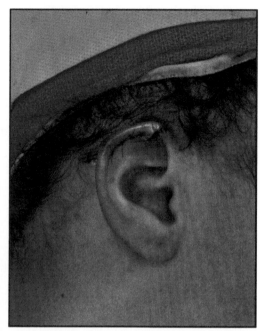

Fig. 78. Final suturing of a defect after a dog bite on the right helix and antihelix in an 8-year-old girl.

SUMMARY

Basic flap design utilization for reconstruction of head and neck defects requires creativity from the surgeon. It is a puzzle with multiple correct solutions. Ultimately, the surgeon must closely restore the basic functions and properties of the surgical flap and adjacent tissue. All options within the reconstructive ladder should be considered. When possible, like should be replaced with like (similar tissue) within an esthetic zone. When considering a flap design, the surgeon must remember that the donor site must be closed in an esthetic and functional manner. Finally, knowledge of normal anatomy, the extent of the defect, and the patient is pivotal for successful outcomes.

REFERENCES

1. Baker S. Resurfacing flaps in reconstructive rhinoplasty. Aesthetic Plast Surg 2002;26:S17.
2. Baker S. Local cutaneous flaps. Otolaryngol Clin North Am 1994;27:139–59.
3. Baker S. Regional flaps in facial reconstruction. Otolaryngol Clin North Am 1990;23:925–46.
4. Kruger E. Reconstruction of bone and soft tissue in extensive facial defects. J Oral Maxillofac Surg 1982;40:714–20.
5. Escobar V, Zide M. Delayed repair of skin cancer defects. J Oral Maxillofac Surg 1999;57:271–9.
6. Baker S. Local flaps in facial reconstruction. 2nd edition. St Louis (MO): Mosby, Elevier; 2007.
7. Murakami C, Nishioka G. Essential concepts in the design of local skin flaps. Facial Plast Surg Clin North Am 1996;4:455–68.
8. Papel I. Facial plastic and reconstructive surgery. 2nd edition. New York: Thieme Medical Publishers; 2002.
9. Patel KG, Sykes JM. Concepts in local flap design and classification. Operative Techniques in Otolaryngology-Head and Neck Surgery 2011;22:13–23.
10. Gorney M. Tissue dynamics and surgical geometry. Biological aspects of reconstructive surgery. Boston: Little and Brown; 1977.
11. Whiteker D. Rotation pattern flaps. In: Wheeland R, editor. Cutaneous surgery. Philadelphia: Saunders; 1994.
12. Bray D. Rhomboc flaps. In: Baker S, Swanson N, editors. Local flaps in facial reconstruction. St Louis (MO): Mosby; 1995. p. 151–63.
13. Zide M, Fuselier C. The partial-thickness cross-lip flap for correction of postoncologic surgical defects. J Oral Maxillofac Surg 2001;59:760–7.
14. Yih W, Howerton D. A regional approach to reconstruction of the upper lip. J Oral Maxillofac Surg 1997;55:383–9.
15. Schulte D, Sherris D, Kasperbaurer J. The anatomical basis of the Abbe flap. Laryngoscope 2001;111:382–6.
16. Massengill R, Pickrell K, Mladick R. Lingual flaps: effect on speech articulation and physiology. Ann Otol Rhinol Laryngol 1970;179:853–7.
17. Tscholi M, Hoy E, Granick M. Skin flaps. Periop Nurs Clin 2011;6:171–86.

Palatal Flap

Jason A. Jamali, DDS, MD

KEYWORDS

- Palatal rotation-advancement flap • Palatal island flap • Reconstruction • Treatment • Defect

KEY POINTS

- The palatal flap offers a technically simple and predictable option for oral reconstruction.
- Palatal flap can be raised as an axial flap (palatal island flap) or random flap (rotation-advancement flap).
- The palatal island modification allows for increased flexibility of flap rotation and decreases the amount of denuded palatal bone at the donor site.
- 75% of the palatal mucosa can be used for closure of defects of up to 16 cm^2.
- Palatal flap can be used alone for simple local reconstruction or together with other regional or free flap for complex reconstruction.

INTRODUCTION

The esthetic and functional demands of maxillofacial reconstruction have driven the evolution of an array of options. Among the various options, it is important that selection takes into account what is most reliable and safest for the patient. Maxillofacial reconstruction can involve local tissue rearrangement and regional flaps. The closer the flap donor site is to the defect, the less morbidity is associated with the reconstructive surgery. Flaps from local tissue also carry the advantages of having similar color and texture. Therefore, the palatal island flap remains popular in reconstructing intraoral defects; moreover, the palatal island flap is the only available flap that can provide keratinized mucosa for defect reconstruction.

The palatal flap was initially described in 1922 by Victor Veau[1] to address oronasal fistulas associated with cleft repair. It was later popularized by Millard[2] for palatal lengthening during cleft repair in the 1960s; however, it was Gullane and Arena[3] who used the flap for postablative defects. The versatility of the palatal island flap led to its widespread use in the 1970s and 1980s; several modifications have been proposed to expand its indications and improve donor site morbidity. Early publications have focused on its use in cleft repair and the closure of oroantral fistulas. Recent publications have shifted the focus to postablative reconstruction, either by itself or together with other flaps.[4]

ANATOMY

The palatal mucosa is strongly adhered to the underlying periosteum, which is subsequently attached to the bone via fibrous tissue pegs known as Sharpey fibers. The osteology of the hard palate is comprised of the palatine process of the maxilla, separated from the horizontal palatal lamina of the palatine bones by a transverse suture. A longitudinal suture separates the maxilla in the midline; the palatal aponeurosis attaches to the posterior margin of the hard palate and is continuous with the tensor veli palatini laterally. The tensor veli palatine muscle arises from the lateral wall of the eustachian tube cartilage, and between the sphenoid spine/scaphoid fossa, before coursing at a right angle anterior to the hamulus to attach to the aponeurosis. The levator veli palatine muscle

Disclosures: None.
Department of Oral and Maxillofacial Surgery, University of Illinois Chicago, 801 South Paulina (MC 835), Chicago, IL 60612, USA
E-mail address: jjamali@uic.edu

Oral Maxillofacial Surg Clin N Am 26 (2014) 305–311
http://dx.doi.org/10.1016/j.coms.2014.05.012
1042-3699/14/$ – see front matter © 2014 Elsevier Inc. All rights reserved.

also meets in the midline, with fibers inserting into the palatine aponeurosis.

The blood supply arises from the greater palatine foramen adjacent to the maxillary second molar, where the transverse suture divides the maxillary and palatal shelves. The descending palatal artery emerges as the greater palatine artery after its exit from the foramen. It eventually anastomoses anteriorly with the nasopalatine branch of the sphenopalatine artery. A rich anastomotic network exists between the right and left greater palatine arteries, exiting across the midline longitudinal raphe. This network, which courses within the mucosa, submucosa, and periosteum, is referred to as a "trilaminar macronet."[5] As a result of this dense network, the entire hard palate mucosa can be elevated on a single neurovascular pedicle. Posteriorly, greater palatine artery also demonstrates a great vascular network with the ascending pharyngeal artery in the soft palate.[6] This rich vascular network allows the flap to be raised as a random flap even in the case of greater palatine artery ligation.[7] With regard to drainage, the veins empty into the pterygoid or pharyngeal venous plexus.

INDICATIONS AND CONTRAINDICATIONS

The defect location and size determine the available reconstructive options. As an axial flap, the palatal flap is limited in the extent of its range; however, it has been applied to oropharyngeal defects, which include the retromolar trigone,[8] soft palate,[9,10] tonsillar fossa,[11] cheek,[12,13] posterior one-third of the floor of the mouth,[14,15] and oronasal and oroantral fistula closures.[16–21] With regard to defect size, up to 75% of the palatal mucosa may be used, allowing defects of up to 16 cm^2 to be closed.[22] However, when harvested as a random flap, the palatal flap is more suitable for oral-antral/nasal communication. Because of the less reliable vascular blood supply, a palatal flap harvested in a random pattern should not cross the midline and maintain the length/width ratio at less than 2.4:1.[7]

The flap is contraindicated whenever there is concern for a compromised blood supply. This may result from a history of ipsilateral internal carotid artery ligation, surgeries with adjacent incisions, or radiation therapy, which have been shown to increase the risk of flap failure.[3] Although prior histories of vessel ligation or palatal surgery are uncommon, radiation to the palate is commonly encountered in patients with oropharyngeal cancer. Additionally, in children less than 5 years of age, concerns regarding iatrogenic midface growth restriction limit its use.[4]

TECHNIQUE

The patient is prepared and draped in regular oral and maxillofacial surgical fashion. Oral intubation with the placement of a Dingmen retractor is usually recommended to facilitate the surgery. Important flap landmarks include (1) palatal gingival crest, (2) greater palatal foremen (palatal to the maxillary second molar), (3) boundary between hard and soft palate, and (4) hamular notch.

The flap design begins after confirming the dimensions of the defect. The anterior region of the flap should be slightly wider than the defect, and the length should allow for a tension-free closure. A template can be trimmed to the dimensions of the defect to help with flap design, whereas the lateral incision is made approximately 5 mm from the gingival margins of the teeth, if present (**Figs. 1** and **2**). After full-thickness incisions are made through the mucoperiosteum, flap dissection proceeds from anterior to posterior, working toward the neurovascular bundle ipsilateral side, and requires ligation of the contralateral neurovascular bundle in addition to the incisal canal (**Fig. 3**). After raising the flap, the neurovascular bundle is dissected carefully from the undersurface of the proximal portion of the flap. The dissection continues until the distal portion of the flap being used for the defect is encountered. Finally, the mucosa is transected above the bundle, allowing for and leaving the remaining distal end of the mucosa attached to the bundle. The bundle may be tunneled under adjacent mucosa before reaching the intended defect; however, care must be taken to ensure there is no compression (**Fig. 4**). Alternatively, the pedicle can cross over the normal palatal tissue before reaching the reconstruction site. This alternative requires second-stage surgery, which can be undertaken approximately 3 weeks later.[13]

In some instances, additional length may be needed to ensure a tension-free closure. This

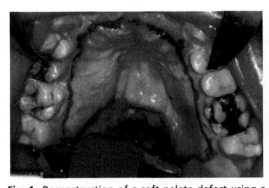

Fig. 1. Reconstruction of a soft palate defect using a palatal rotation flap. (*Courtesy of* Drs Joseph Helman and Brent B. Ward, Ann Arbor, MI.)

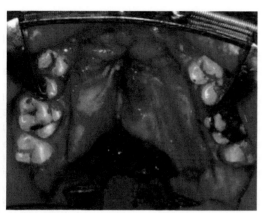

Fig. 2. Outlining the margins of the flap. (*Courtesy of* Drs Joseph Helman and Brent B. Ward, Ann Arbor, MI.)

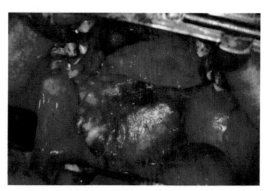

Fig. 4. Flap sutured in place. (*Courtesy of* Drs Joseph Helman and Brent B. Ward, Ann Arbor, MI.)

may be accomplished through decompression of the posterior wall of the greater palatine foramen and fracture of the hamulus. In some instances, up to 1 cm of additional length can be gained when using this technique.[15]

After the defect closure, the denuded bone may be addressed using either iodoform gauze sutured in place or a preformed stent. When using a stent, it is important to ensure that there is no pedicle compression. Re-epithelialization may take between 3 and 5 weeks, although in smokers this may be delayed to 6 to 8 weeks (**Fig. 5**).

Although morbidity is relatively low in the donor site, the patients should be instructed to maintain excellent oral hygiene and eliminate cigarette smoking until the wounds are healed. Postoperative chlorhexidine mouthwash is often prescribed.

Modifications

Random rotation-advancement flap
Alternatively, the palatal flap can be raised as a random rotation-advancement flap. Mercer and Maccarthy[6] demonstrated the collateral blood supply between the greater palatine artery and the ascending palatine artery in the soft palate.

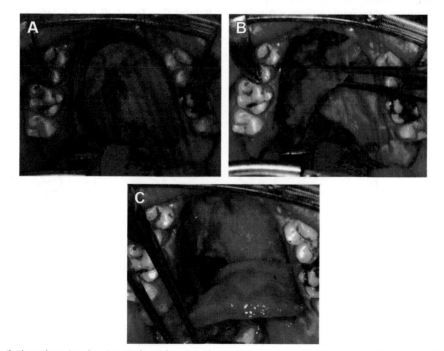

Fig. 3. (*A–C*) Flap elevation begins at the side contralateral to the pedicle. (*Courtesy of* Drs Joseph Helman and Brent B. Ward, Ann Arbor, MI.)

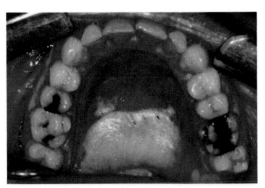

Fig. 5. At 6-week follow-up with epithelialization of the denuded bone. (*Courtesy of* Drs Joseph Helman and Brent B. Ward, Ann Arbor, MI.)

This anatomic basis allows one to sacrifice the greater palatine artery without jeopardizing the vitality of the flap.[7] The flap is raised similarly to its axial counterpart; however, no incision is made in the proximal end of this flap, and the medial aspect of the flap does not cross the midline (2–3 mm away from the midline). This modification of the flap has a limited arc of rotation; therefore, it is more commonly used for closure of oral-antral or oral-nasal fistulas (**Fig. 6**).[20] Unlike other techniques in closing oral-antral/nasal fistulas, which require at least two-layer closures, the palatal flap can close the communication in a single layer.[16–21]

The palatal flap can also be raised as an anterior-based random rotation-advancement flap. In this scenario, the distal portion of the flap is left intact to maintain its vascularity. Similar to its posterior-based counterpart, the mobility of this flap is limited and mainly used for fistula closure.

Submucosal modification

A conventional palatal flap leaves the donor site with a denuded palatal bone, which can create great discomfort for the patients. Alternatively, Yamazaki and colleagues[23] proposed a submucosal variance of the flap. In this modification, the submucosal palatal tissue is separated from the superficial layer, and dissected off the palatal bone. The flap can be raised as either axial or random flaps, and once the flap has been raised, the superficial layer is reapproximated to provide palatal coverage. This modification helps to relieve the postoperative discomfort that patients might encounter with the conventional technique. Unfortunately, few have advocated its use because of limited benefits and technical challenge in maintaining the integrity of the superficial layer during dissection. However, a variation of this flap, the vascularized interpositional periosteal-connective tissue flap,[24–26] has been popularized in the practice of implant dentistry. Vascularized interpositional periosteal-connective tissue is an anteriorly based random pattern submucosal palatal rotational flap (**Fig. 7**). It is commonly used to reconstruct soft tissue defects in the anterior maxilla, such as soft tissue augmentation in implant dentistry[24,25] or soft tissue coverage in the alveolar cleft.[26]

Palatal flap for skull-based defects

The advancements in endoscopic surgery provide a treatment alternative for skull-based tumors;

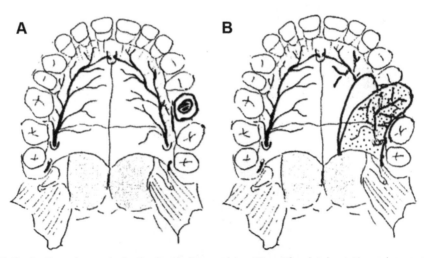

Fig. 6. (*A, B*) Illustrations demonstrate the harvesting and insetting of palatal rotation-advancement flap for closure of oral-antral communication. (*From* Anavi Y, Gavriel G, Silfen R, et al. Palatal rotation-advancement flap for delayed repair of oroantral fistula: a retrospective evaluation of 63 Cases. Oral Surg Oral Med Oral Pathol Oral Radiol Endod 2003;96(5):529; with permission from Elsevier.)

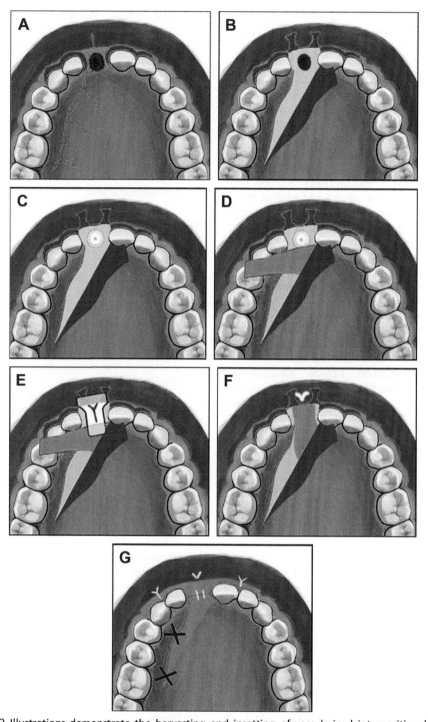

Fig. 7. (*A–G*) Illustrations demonstrate the harvesting and insetting of vascularized interpositional periosteal-connective tissue flap for dental implant in the anterior maxilla. (*From* Kim CS, Jang YJ, Choi SH, et al. Long-term results from soft and hard tissue augmentation by a modified vascularized interpositional periosteal-connective tissue technique in the maxillary anterior region. J Oral Maxillofac Surg 2012;70(2):484–91; with permission.)

however, endoscopic skull-based surgery is limited by its reconstructive options. Most reconstruction options in this surgery rely on local flaps or artificial grafts, and both of these options are limited by their size and vitality. Oliver and colleagues[27–29] were the first to propose the use of an axial palatal island flap to reconstruct skull-based defects after endoscopic surgery. This flap provides a large surface area (12–18.5 cm^2) and adequate pedicle length (29.1 mm) to reconstruct most skull-based defects.

Complications

The palatal flap has relatively few postoperative complications, and the flap failure rate is low when it is harvested in an axial pattern. Gullane and Arena[3] reported a failure rate of 5% in the axial pattern palatal flap, and from their 53 case-series, the factors associated with flap failure included a history of head and neck radiation, prior ligation of the external carotid and internal maxillary artery, and previous palatal surgery. Although seldom reported, Urken[22] warned of possible flap necrosis caused by excessive tension on the artery, as a result of its vessel course through the bony canal.

When the palatal flap was harvested as a random flap, the failure rate increased to 25%. Lee and colleagues[7] emphasized the importance of the length/width ratio in the survival of a random palatal flap; a length/width ratio greater than 2.4:1 is associated with significant flap failure.

Other complications include intraoperative bleeding caused by injury to the greater palatine vessels, or in some cases, a secondary major vessel, which came out of the minor palatine foramen.[4] Hemostasis can usually be obtained with pressure and meticulous cautery. An injury to the greater palatine artery does not lead to aborting the procedure automatically, as long as the proximal portion of the palatal mucosa has not yet been incised. This flap can still survive as a random rotation-advancement flap.[7]

DISCUSSION

For oropharyngeal reconstruction, the goal is to satisfy form (adequate thickness, pliability, and so forth) and function (speech, swallowing, and so forth), while minimizing donor site morbidity, operative risk, and time. Oropharyngeal reconstruction can be accomplished using grafts, obturator placement, or microvascular tissue transfer. Although microvascular techniques can provide a greater volume of tissue, in general, they require increased operative time, donor site morbidity, recovery time, and in some instances debulking. Obturators offer decreased operative time and no donor site morbidity; however, retention of the prosthesis may be problematic, and speech and swallowing deficits may persist.

For a small defect, palatal flap can provide a simple solution to a difficult problem. For a complex defect (ie, through-and-through defect), palatal flap has been used together with either free or local flaps. For example, the addition of the palatal rotational flap to myomucosal pharyngeal constrictor advancement flaps[15] can provide increased rigidity; or the free fasciocutaneous flap for complex oromandibular reconstruction.[23]

The palatal flap offers a technically simple and predictable option for intraoral reconstruction. The patients usually encounter minimal postoperative morbidity, and should expect a rapid return to a normal diet. Although the palatal flap cannot serve as a panacea for most intraoral reconstruction, it provides the reconstructive surgeon with a great armamentarium.

REFERENCES

1. Division Palatine: Anatomie—chirurgie Phonétique. By Victor Veau, Chirurgien De l'Hôpital Des Enfants Assistés, with the Collaboration of Mme. S. Borel. Large 8vo. Pp. 568 Viii, with 786 Illustrations. 1931. Paris: Masson Et Cie. Fr. 140.
2. Millard DR. A new use of the island flap in wide palate clefts. Plast Reconstr Surg 1966;38(4):330–5.
3. Gullane PJ, Arena S. Palatal island flap for reconstruction of oral defects. Arch Otolaryngol 1977; 103(10):598–9.
4. Seckel NG. The palatal island flap on retrospection. Plast Reconstr Surg 1995;96(6):1262–8.
5. Maher WP. Distribution of palatal and other arteries in cleft and non-cleft human palates. Cleft Palate J 1977;14(1):1–12.
6. Mercer NS, Maccarthy P. The arterial supply of the palate. Plast Reconstr Surg 1995;96(5):1038–44.
7. Lee JJ, Kok SH, Chang HH, et al. Repair of oroantral communications in the third molar region by random palatal flap. Int J Oral Maxillofac Surg 2002;31(6): 677–80.
8. Genden EM, Lee BB, Urken ML. The palatal island flap for reconstruction of palatal and retromolar trigone defects revisited. Arch Otolaryngol Head Neck Surg 2001;127(7):827–41.
9. Karle WE, Anand SM, Clain JB, et al. Total soft palate reconstruction using the palatal island and lateral pharyngeal wall flaps. Laryngoscope 2013;123(4): 929–33.
10. Moore BA, Magdy E, Netterville JL, et al. Palatal reconstruction with the palatal island flap. Laryngoscope 2003;113(6):946–51.
11. Magdy EA. The palatal island mucoperiosteal flap for primary intraoral reconstruction following tumor ablative surgery. Eur Arch Otorhinolaryngol 2011; 268(11):1633–8.
12. Mehrotra D, Pradhan R, Gupta S. Retrospective comparison of surgical treatment modalities in 100 patients with oral submucous fibrosis. Oral Surg Oral Med Oral Pathol Oral Radiol Endod 2009; 107(3):E1–10.

13. Khanna JN, Andrade NN. Oral submucous fibrosis: a new concept in surgical management. Int J Oral Maxillofac Surg 1995;24(6):433–9.
14. Komisar A, Lawson W. A compendium of intraoral flaps. Head Neck Surg 1985;8(2):91–9.
15. Ward BB. The palatal flap. Oral Maxillofac Surg Clin North Am 2003;15(4):467–73.
16. Visscher SH, Van Minnen B, Bos RR. Closure of oroantral communications: a review of the literature. J Oral Maxillofac Surg 2010;68(6):1384–91.
17. Garner JM, Wein RO. Use of the palatal flap for closure of an oronasal fistula. Am J Otolaryngol 2006;27(4):268–70.
18. Yalçın S, Öncü B, Emes Y, et al. Surgical treatment of oroantral fistulas: a clinical study of 23 cases. J Oral Maxillofac Surg 2011;69(2):333–9.
19. Lehman JA. Closure of palatal fistulas. Operat Tech Plast Reconstr Surg 1995;2(4):255–62.
20. Anavi Y, Gal G, Silfen R, et al. Palatal rotation-advancement flap for delayed repair of oroantral fistula: a retrospective evaluation of 63 cases. Oral Surg Oral Med Oral Pathol Oral Radiol Endod 2003;96(5):527–34.
21. Abuabara A, Cortez AL, Passeri LA, et al. Evaluation of different treatments for oroantral/oronasal communications: experience of 112 cases. Int J Oral Maxillofac Surg 2006;35(2):155–8.
22. Urken ML. "Palatal island." Atlas of regional and free flaps for head and neck reconstruction: flap harvest and insetting. 2nd edition. Philadelphia: Wolters Kluwer Health/Lippincott Williams & Wilkins; 2012. p. 130–7.
23. Yamazaki Y, Yamaoka M, Hirayama M, et al. The submucosal island flap in the closure of oro-antral fistula. Br J Oral Maxillofac Surg 1985;23(4):259–63.
24. Sclar A. The vascularized interpositional periosteal-connective tissue (VIP-CT) flap. In: Sclar A, editor. Soft tissue and esthetic considerations in implant therapy. Chicago: Quintessence Publishing; 2003. p. 163–87.
25. Kim CS, Jang YJ, Choi SH, et al. Long-term results from soft and hard tissue augmentation by a modified vascularized interpositional periosteal-connective tissue technique in the maxillary anterior region. J Oral Maxillofac Surg 2012;70(2):484–91.
26. Rahpeyma A, Khajehahmadi S. Modified VIP-CT flap in late maxillary alveolar cleft surgery. J Craniomaxillofac Surg 2014;42(5):432–7.
27. Oliver CL, Hackman TG, Carrau RL, et al. Palatal flap modifications allow pedicled reconstruction of the skull base. Laryngoscope 2008;118(12):2102–6.
28. Hackman T, Chicoine MR, Uppaluri R. Novel application of the palatal island flap for endoscopic skull base reconstruction. Laryngoscope 2009;119(8):1463–6.
29. Ducic Y, Herford AS. The use of palatal island flaps as an adjunct to microvascular free tissue transfer for reconstruction of complex oromandibular defects. Laryngoscope 2001;111(9):1666–9.

Tongue Flaps

Robert A. Strauss, DDS, MD*, Nicholas J. Kain, DDS

KEYWORDS

- Tongue flap • Flap reconstruction • Oral and maxillofacial surgery

KEY POINTS

- Although limited to anatomic defects located within a short arc of rotation, the dorsal or lateral tongue flap, when indicated, is a safe, reliable, and low-morbidity reconstructive option.
- The dorsal or lateral tongue flap is particularly useful for defects in the palate, floor of mouth, pharynx, and buccal mucosa.
- Complications are rare and usually minor. It is imperative, however, that a well thought out strategy for airway management is planned, especially for the second-stage procedure.

INTRODUCTION AND HISTORY

Historically, intraoral flap reconstruction in oral and maxillofacial surgery (OMS) primarily involved simple buccal or palatal sliding flaps to cover oral-antral fistulas or an occasional intraoral small bone graft. Over the past decade, however, the specialty of OMS has evolved and expanded the wide range of procedures and diseases that are treated on a daily basis that necessitate soft tissue coverage. The ever-increasing use and sophistication of dental implants require equally sophisticated local soft tissue management, and the greater involvement of the OMS in the extirpation and reconstruction of cancer has led down the path of distant flap transfer and microvascular free tissue flaps. At the same time, new or newly recognized conditions, such as osteoradionecrosis and bisphosphonate-related osteonecrosis of the jaws, have created a new population of patients needing complex tissue coverage.

As the number of procedures needed has increased, so have the variety and complexity of possible flap designs. An ideal flap would be simple to perform in an office or as an outpatient procedure, have little down time for patients, have minimal complications, and provide ample and supple tissue to any area of the mouth or face as needed. Although no perfect flap exists to date, the tongue flap meets many of these criteria and has, over time, proved a utilitarian, reliable flap that can be used in many common defects. In addition, unlike many of the distant and microvascular flaps that require additional subspecialized or fellowship training, the tongue flap is well within the scope of practice and training of just about any practicing oral and maxillofacial surgeon, not only related to the procedure itself but also the management of its few potential complications.

Although the tongue flap seemingly is currently having resurgence in popularity, it is not a new procedure. The procedure was first described more than 100 years ago, initially by Eiselsberg for intraoral defects and soon after by Lexer, who described its use for defects of the retromolar trigone and tonsillar areas.[1,2] Technical difficulties precluded its widespread use until several articles in the 1950s and 1960s described technical advancements that made this flap a useful and viable tool to manage closure of palatal defects and oral-antral fistulas.[3] Since that time, there have been many articles describing the use of this flap in its various formats (lateral, dorsal, anterior based, posterior based, and so forth) for transposition into a variety of defects.

Department of Oral and Facial Surgery, Virginia Commonwealth University Medical Center, PO Box 980566, Richmond, VA 23298, USA
* Corresponding author.
E-mail address: rastrauss@vcu.edu

Oral Maxillofacial Surg Clin N Am 26 (2014) 313–325
http://dx.doi.org/10.1016/j.coms.2014.05.002

APPLIED SURGICAL ANATOMY

The tongue is a muscular hydrostat (functional muscular tissue without skeletal support) formed by a mass of skeletal muscle covered with keratinized stratified squamous epithelium. On average, the tongue is 12 to 14 cm in length.[4] Embryologically, the tongue is formed from components of the first 4 pharyngeal arches. The anterior two-thirds of the tongue lie in the oral cavity and are derived from the first pharyngeal arch, whereas the posterior third is contained in the oropharynx and hypopharynx and is derived from the third pharyngeal arch.[5] The tongue functions in deglutition (swallowing), mastication (chewing), gustation (tasting), and phonation (vocalization).

The tongue is divided into right and left halves by a median fibrous septum. The muscles of the tongue are attached to the hyoid bone, mandible, styloid process, palate, and pharynx. The tongue musculature is divided into 4 intrinsic and 4 extrinsic muscles. All the tongue muscles are innervated by the hypoglossal nerve (cranial nerve XII), except for the palatoglossus muscle, which is innervated by the pharyngeal plexus of the vagus nerve (cranial nerve X). The intrinsic muscles of the tongue are used to change the shape of the tongue and do not attach to bone or aid in movement. The intrinsic tongue muscles include the superior longitudinalis, the inferior longitudinalis, the transversus, and the verticalis muscles. The extrinsic muscles of the tongue all originate from bone and function to allow tongue movement. The extrinsic tongue muscles include the genioglossus, the hyoglossus, the styloglossus, and the palatoglossus muscles.[5,6]

The anterior and posterior parts of tongue are separated by the V-shaped sulcus terminalis. The foramen cecum is located in the midline, approximately 2.5 cm anterior to the tongue base, at the junction of the 2 arms of the sulcus terminalis. Neurologically, the general somatic afferent innervation to the anterior two-thirds of the tongue is via the lingual branch of the third division of the trigeminal nerve (cranial nerve V), and taste sensation is via the chorda tympani, which is a branch of the facial nerve (cranial nerve VII) traveling with the lingual nerve. The general visceral afferent innervation and taste sensation to the posterior third of the tongue are supplied via the glossopharyngeal nerve (cranial nerve IX).[5,6]

The blood supply of the tongue is supplied via the lingual artery, the tonsillar branch of the facial artery, and the ascending pharyngeal artery. The vast majority of the blood supply of the tongue is via the lingual artery, which is the third direct branch of the external carotid artery. The lingual artery arises from the anterior surface of the external carotid artery at the level of the greater horn of the hyoid bone in the Pirogoff triangle (formed by the intermediate tendon of the digastric muscle, the posterior border of the mylohyoid muscle, and the hypoglossal nerve). The anatomic location of the lingual artery has also be described using the Lesser triangle (formed by the hypoglossal nerve and the anterior and posterior bellies of the digastric muscle), with the artery lying within the triangle deep to the hyoglossus muscle. Access to the Pirogoff and Lesser triangles is clinically important because they allow for ligation of the most proximal trunk of the lingual artery. The lingual artery passes deep to the hyoglossus muscle and lies on the middle pharyngeal constrictor as it advances into the posterior lateral tongue. The lingual artery gives rise to the suprahyoid artery, the dorsal lingual artery, the sublingual artery, and the deep lingual artery. The suprahyoid artery travels along the superior border of the hyoid bone and supplies the suprahyoid musculature. The dorsal lingual artery arises caudal to the hyoglossus muscle and supplies the dorsum of the tongue, the vallecula, tonsils, glossopalatine arch, and the adjacent soft palate. In the tip of the tongue, the ranine branch anastomoses the bilateral dorsal lingual arteries into a rich plexus. The sublingual artery arises at the anterior border of the hyoglossus muscle and travels along the genioglossus muscle and sublingual gland toward the midline where it anastomosis with the opposite side. The sublingual artery supplies the mylohyoid muscle, the sublingual gland, the floor of the mouth, and the lingual mandibular alveolus and gingiva. It also has a branch that pierces the mylohyoid muscle and anastomoses with the ipsilateral facial artery. The deep lingual artery is the terminal branch of the lingual artery, which travels a torturous course along the ventral surface of the tongue lying on the inferior side of the inferior longitudinalis muscle, the lateral surface of the genioglossus muscle, and just deep to the ventral mucosa toward the tip of the tongue. After traversing the hyoglossus muscle, the deep lingual artery travels with the lingual nerve. The bilateral deep lingual arteries anastomose posteriorly via the transverse lingual artery and at the tip of the tongue via a large anastomotic plexus.[5,6] Clinically, the rich anastomotic plexuses formed between the branches of the bilateral lingual arteries make hemorrhage control difficult with only unilateral lingual artery ligation.

The paired lingual veins are formed from the tributaries of the deep lingual veins, sublingual veins, suprahyoid veins, and the dorsal lingual veins. The lingual veins drain directly into the internal jugular veins. The vena comitans of the hypoglossal nerve, also known as the ranine vein, begins at the tip of the tongue and travels along the course of the hypoglossal nerve. The ranine vein either empties into the lingual vein or the common facial vein.[5,6]

The lymphatic drainage from the tip of the tongue drains into the submental lymph nodes. The remainder of the anterior two-thirds of the tongue drains into the submandibular and deep cervical lymph nodes. The posterior third of the tongue drains in the deep cervical lymph nodes.[5,6] These lymphatic drainage pathways are important to consider when managing malignancies of the tongue.

INDICATIONS, CONTRAINDICATIONS, ALTERNATIVES
Indications

The tongue flap is an extremely versatile flap that can be used for the reconstruction of many oral, pharyngeal, and perioral defects. Depending on the type of tongue flap used, congenital, ablative, or traumatic defects of the lip; commissure; buccal mucosa; palate; alveolus; tongue; floor of mouth; or pharynx can be adequately reconstructed.

One frequently used application of the tongue flap is closure of oronasal and oroantral communications and fistulas that have failed reconstructive therapy with local advancement or rotational mucoperiosteal flaps. Oronasal fistulas commonly form in the midline or paramedian hard palate secondary to breakdown of repaired palatal clefts, from traumatic injuries or pathologic excision. These defects can propose a significant reconstructive challenge, that in many cases can prove refractory to conventional therapy, due to the defect size, scarring, or lack of adequate local soft tissue. Depending on the anatomic position of the oronasal fistula, anterior- or posterior-based dorsal tongue flaps can be used to successfully reconstruct the fistula. When a surgeon prefers a 2-layer closure, the tongue flap can be combined with hinged mucoperiosteal flaps from the fistula periphery or vomer flaps to create a nasal floor and layered closure of the fistula (Fig. 1).[7] The dorsal tongue flap should be designed to be approximately 20% larger than the defect to compensate for flap contracture, and the paddle can be specifically shaped to adapt to the individualized defect contours.[8,9] Morel and colleagues[10] have shown excellent results when applying the lateral tongue flap to cleft palate defects. When oroantral fistulas are too large for treatment with, or fail, traditional closure with mucoperiosteal advancement flaps (with or without

buccal fat pad grafts), lateral tongue flaps have been used with success.[11]

Tongue flaps can also be used for the reconstruction of posttraumatic defects, postablative defects, and syndromic hypoplasia of the upper and lower lips. The tongue flap for lip reconstruction has shown good long-term functional and esthetic results with no major complications, minimal flap necrosis secondary to the abundant blood supply, and only temporary speech and masticatory interruption.[12] Lateral, dorsal, or ventral tongue flaps can be used alone or in conjuncture with other local and free flaps, based on the size and location of the lip defect.[13–16] The anterior-based ventral surface myomucosal tongue flap has been shown to adequately restore the form and function of the lip commissure secondary to electrical burns. The tongue myomucosal flap helps relieve the scar contracture through composite replacement of the skin, mucosa, and orbicularis oris muscle. This improves lip mobility, facial expression, and oral competence.[17] The anterior-based ventral surface tongue flap has also been shown to simultaneously reconstruct the lower lip mucosal surface and vermillion, with the addition of lower lip bulk and without obliteration of the vestibule.[18] Ventral tongue mucosal or myomucosal flaps have been used to reconstruct the vermillion border after lip shave procedures for squamous cell carcinoma and veruccous carcinoma with excellent esthetic results.[19] Lateral and ventral tongue flaps have been used to reconstruct the hypoplastic vermillion and lip defects secondary to Parry-Romberg syndrome. The ventral tongue flap has the advantage of lacking papilla to allow for a more conspicuous vermillion border reconstruction. The main disadvantage of the tongue flap for lip and vermillion reconstruction is the potential for color mismatch, especially in racially pigmented lips.[20]

Due to surgical ease, tongue flap reconstruction of buccal mucosal defects is performed most commonly using the double-door flap technique, where a horizontal incision along the lateral border of the tongue allows for the creation of a superior and inferior myomucosal flap used to cover the defect.[1] Lateral-based tongue flaps can also be used to reconstruct buccal mucosal defects and have been shown a simple, effective, salvage reconstructive option in previously radiated patients where microvascular free tissue transfer is not an option.[21] The tongue flap has shown promising results as an adjunct for reconstruction of buccal mucosal stricture secondary to oral submucous fibrosis with similar results in postoperative mouth opening compared with buccal fat pad grafts, nasolabial fold flaps, and split-thickness skin grafts.[22]

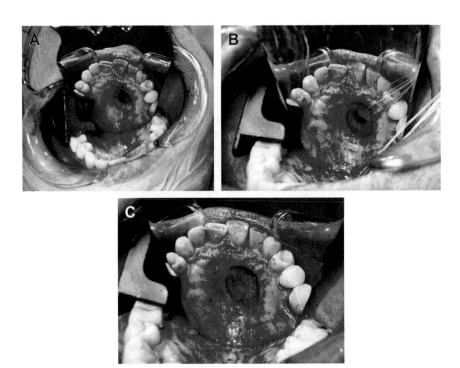

Fig. 1. Incision design for development of hinged mucoperiosteal flap (*A*). Passing of sutures for closure (*B*). Flaps rotated and closed to create nasal floor (*C*).

Sliding and island tongue flaps can be used to reconstruct both anterior and posterior tongue defects. Small tongue defects (<1/4) can be closed primarily with minimal associated morbidity, but medium- and large-sized defects can cause significant problems with tongue mobility if closed primarily or left to heal by secondary intent. It has been shown that with medium-sized tongue defects (4–6 cm in diameter), tongue base island flaps, and sliding posterior tongue flaps can be advanced for closure. This allows for good objective and subjective speech, deglutination, and esthetics.[23,24] Similarly, posterior and base of tongue defects can be reconstructed with anterior-based set back tongue flaps while maintaining near-normal tongue mobility and length.[4,25]

Floor of mouth defects have been successfully reconstructed with the creation of median and paramedian dorsal tongue myomucosal island flaps that are transited through a tunnel in the tongue to allow the paddle to reach to the contralateral sublingual area for coverage with no speech or deglutition disturbances.[26,27] Anteriolateral ventral tongue flaps have also been used with success in reconstructing floor of mouth defects without complication.[28]

Pharyngeal reconstruction using tongue flaps after ablative surgery has been reported for defects up to 8 cm in size with minimal reduction in deglutination. One-third tongue flaps, one-half tongue base flaps, complete tongue base flaps, and transverse tongue base flaps have been described for use alone and in combination with dermal grafts for hypopharynx reconstruction.[29,30]

Contraindications

Contraindications to the use of a tongue flaps for reconstructive surgeries are limited. Patients with severe systemic medical conditions precluding the use of general anesthesia or major reconstructive surgery are generally contraindicated. Patients with psychiatric disorders or developmental delays may be a contraindication due to lack of compliance during the perioperative period, increasing the incidence of flap disruption and failure. Small defects that can be closed primarily or with a skin graft, as well as superficial defects that can heal by secondary intent, are contraindicated for tongue flap reconstruction due to the potential for increased morbidity. Conversely, large defects that are larger than the total surface area obtainable with the tongue flap paddle are contraindicated for this reconstruction. Patients who have previously undergone tongue and/or floor of mouth surgery may be problematic due to lack of tissue volume, limited flap and/or tongue mobility, increased scar tissue, and decreased vascularity. All these can increase the risk of postoperative tongue functional derangement and decrease flap survival due to reduced vascular supply.

Alternatives

There are many local, distant, and free tissue flaps that can be used as alternatives for reconstruction of the oral and perioral defects commonly reconstructed with the tongue flap. These flaps include (but are not limited to) palatal island/finger flaps, buccal mucosal and buccinator muscle flaps, nasolabial flaps, melolabial fold flaps, facial artery myomucosal flaps, buccal fat pad grafts, temporalis muscle flaps, temporoparietal fascia flaps, pectoralis major flap, sternocleidomastoid flaps, platysmal flaps, deltopectoral flaps, trapezius flaps, and a various assortment of microvascular free flaps. Each of these flaps has specific reconstructive indications and contraindications, but discussion of them is beyond the scope of this article.

ANESTHETIC IMPLICATIONS OF TONGUE FLAP SURGERY

The nature of tongue flap surgery creates anesthetic complexity because the procedure disallows easy access to the oral cavity as a route to the airway. Because a vast majority of surgeries using tongue flaps are directly within the airway, the diverse anatomic defects that can be treated by tongue flap, from palatal fistulae in cleft patients to pharyngeal reconstruction, also make each case unique and require great diligence on the part of anesthesiologists.[31]

Because there are 2 distinct procedures associated with a pedicled tongue flap, the inset and the division, each of these presents unique anesthetic issues. The first procedure, to harvest the flap from the tongue and suture it into the defect, is the simpler of the 2 from an anesthetic perspective. Intubation for this procedure is generally via the nasotracheal route and is performed in the standard fashion using direct visual laryngoscopy (DVL). If the flap is performed for correction of a palatal fistula, care must be exercised to not damage the nasal mucosa approximating the fistula. It is the extubation for this portion of the procedure that requires the most attention, because the inserted flap makes reintubation difficult if the airway was compromised at the end of the surgery. In addition, many patients are placed in maxillomandibular fixation (MMF) at the end of the surgery, to limit mouth opening and protect the flap.[32] This contributes to the difficulty of emergent reintubation. Therefore, anesthesiologists must insure

that patients are calm at the conclusion of surgery to minimize trauma to the flap during arousal from anesthesia but must also be assured that the airway is patent and that patients safely maintain ventilation and not require urgent or emergent reintubation. Because of this concern, some investigators have stated that the use of MMF is neither necessary nor indicated after tongue flap.[33,34] If nasal intubation is not possible, the procedure can be accomplished with an oral tube placed to the contralateral side, although this does make the procedure more difficult.

The second surgery, to divide the newly vascularized flap and reinsert the distal aspect into the defect and the proximal aspect back into the tongue (if indicated and desired) is far more challenging for anesthesiologists. If MMF has been applied, the anesthesiologist and the surgeon must concur on the advisability of opening the MMF prior to induction. There are also many other factors that must be considered when creating an anesthetic plan, including age of patients, anatomic site of defect, site of the tongue flap pedicle, and presence or absence of a pharyngeal flap in cleft patients.

In typical patients without a large previous palatoplasty or pharyngeal flap, nasal intubation allows for the best visibility and access and is the preferred approach. DVL, although technically more difficult in the presence of the pedicle, can be performed using a variety of modifications. In many patients, the left molar approach has been found to allow improved visibility.[35] The right molar approach, however, may allow improved visibility in some cases and should be considered. Although the curved MacIntosh laryngoscope blade was recommended by Yamamoto,[35] the use of straight Miller blade has been advocated by some investigators due to its generally diminished cross-sectional width compared with the MacIntosh blade of equal size.[36]

Some modifications to typical intubation also can make the process less traumatic. Because the surgical procedure to divide and inset the flap is usually quick, the use of an endotracheal tube with an internal diameter 0.5 to 1.0 mm less than the typical size facilitates easy passage through the nose without compromising ventilation during this short time period. Using a soft-textured tube that has been soaked in hot water also allows easier passage. Because blind nasal passage of an endotracheal tube could lead to damage to the nasal mucosa or the inset flap, it is advisable to pass a well-lubricated soft suction or nasogastric catheter through the nose into the pharynx first, then advancing the endotracheal tube over the catheter.[37]

Although DVL is possible for second-stage surgery, the use of fiberoptic laryngoscopy is rapidly becoming the gold standard in this case. This not only improves visibility but also allows the endotracheal tube to be passed over the scope to decrease the possibility of damage to the soft tissues. Passing the tube fitted with a Y-shaped bronchoscope adaptor over the scope until it is just above the epiglottis and closing the mouth and nostrils allows for manual or mechanical ventilation (and the administration of an inhalational anesthetic) during the process of passing the scope into the glottis, allowing a controlled and slow intubation while maintaining oxygen saturation (**Fig. 2**). Although fiberoptic intubation is now considered the preferred approach for almost all tongue flap takedowns, this technique requires both equipment and training that is not universally available. Hence, astute anesthesiologists should be familiar with several possible methods to safely manage the airway in these patients.

In general, nasotracheal intubation is preferred over oral intubation for the increased visibility and access afforded by this approach. When the passage of the nasal pathway is not possible, however, due to a large cleft palatoplasty, the presence of a pharyngeal flap in a cleft patent, a nasal malformation, or acomorbid medical condition (eg, hereditary hemorrhagic telangectasia) other options should be entertained.[33] Oral

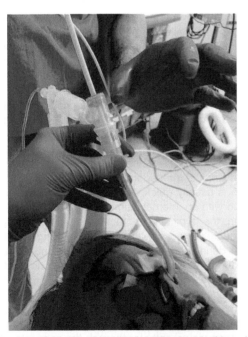

Fig. 2. Y-shaped bronchoscope adaptor in place allowing for ventilation of the patient and simultaneous fiberoptic intubation.

intubation is possible but handicaps surgeons and is difficult for the anesthesiologists. Tracheostomy has been advocated in these cases but seems warranted only in the most severe cases.[38]

Another option is to divide the flap under local anesthesia without vasoconstrictor. This is accomplished by tying 2 silk sutures around the flap and cutting between them. Any bleeding is easily controlled with bipolar cautery. Once this is done, patients can then be intubated for the remainder of the surgery in the standard fashion with care to prevent damage to the flap, which relies on cooperation by patients and may not be suitable in some children.[39]

SURGICAL PROCEDURES
Dorsal Tongue Flap

The dorsal tongue flap is based on the dorsal lingual artery and can be either anterior or posterior based, depending on the location of the defect, and is commonly used for intraoral reconstructive surgery. Defects of the posterior buccal mucosa, retromolar trigone, tonsillar fossa, posterior hard palate, and soft palate are indicated for reconstruction with a posterior-based dorsal tongue flap (**Fig. 3**). Due to the arterial supply to the dorsal tongue feeding from posterior to anterior, posterior-based dorsal tongue flaps have a more robust blood supply, making them more predictable than anterior-based dorsal tongue flaps.[40] Anterior-based dorsal tongue flaps are excellent for reconstruction of the anterior hard palate, anterior buccal mucosa, floor of mouth, and lip/vermillion/commissure defects and are commonly favored for their increased mobility (**Fig. 4**). The dorsal tongue flap should be at least 3 mm thick and include at least a small layer of intrinsic muscle to prevent vascular compromise but should be limited to no more than 10 mm in thickness to prevent undue morbid changes in postoperative tongue function.[41,42] The dorsal tongue flap paddle should be designed to be approximately 20% larger than the defect to account for flap contracture and can be tailored to the shape of the defect.[8,9] A beveled outline of the flap paddle and tip facilitates a smooth primary closure of the donor site.[43] Up to two-thirds of the dorsum of the tongue can be included in the flap without significant deformity.[42] The residual tongue body narrows after flap elevation but does not shorten. The dorsal tongue flap should not be carried posterior to the circumvallate papillae to prevent damage to the feeding vessels.[43,44] The flap length should be appropriate to extend and cover the entire defect but should still allow for tongue mobility. During flap inset, it is important to avoid

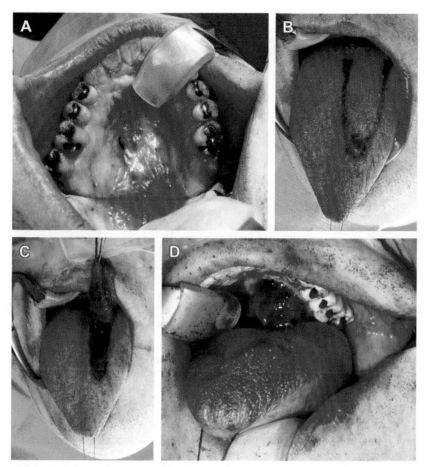

Fig. 3. Oronasal fistula of the posterior lateral hard palate (*A*). Design of posterior-based dorsal tongue flap (*B*). Elevation of flap (*C*). Inset of flap (*D*).

placing any sutures through the muscular flap pedicle, which could strangulate the flap. Any small residual defects left in the area of the proximal pedicle attachment can be easily closed after flap sectioning in the second-stage surgery. If a second-stage procedure is planned, it should be performed after approximately 14 to 21 days of healing to allow for adequate neovascularization and to prevent vascular compromise of the recipient site. The excess flap pedicle can be reinserted into the dorsal surface of the tongue to increase the muscular bulk and prevent postoperative dysfunction and deformity; however, this is often unnecessary.[44] Patients may be kept in maxillomandibular fixation with elastics or wires postoperatively, prior to second-stage surgery, to prevent excessive tongue mobility and the possibility of flap dislodgement or disinsertion. Alternatively, the tongue can be tethered to the floor of the mouth with sutures passing from the submental region through the dorsal tongue. A button can be added to the suture to increase surface area

and prevent the sutures from pulling through the soft tissue. If indicated, debulking and/or recontouring of the inset flap at the recipient site should be delayed for at least 3 months after stage 2 surgery.[9] If a 1-stage procedure is planned, as is the case with laterally positioned defects, the transversed mucosa can be denuded or incised and the entire length of the tongue flap inset. This prevents burying of the traversed mucosa and aids in the blood supply of the flap.[43]

Ventral Tongue Flap

Ventral tongue flaps are anteriorly based and are excellent for reconstruction of the floor of the mouth, the labial surface and vermillion of the lower lip, and the lip commissures. The ventral surface of the tongue has the benefit of not having papilla, making the reconstruction have a more confluent surface color and texture with the surrounding native tissue. The ventral tongue flap can be unilateral or midline based, including tissue

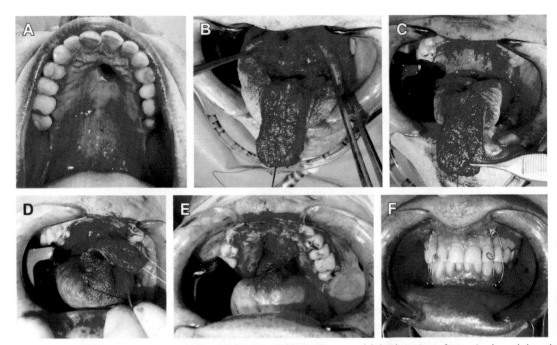

Fig. 4. Oronasal fistula of the anterior hard palate secondary cyst removal (*A*). Elevation of anterior-based dorsal tongue flap (*B*). Closure of the dorsal tongue donor site (*C*). Placement of sutures prior to flap inset (*D*). Final inset of anterior-based dorsal tongue flap into the defect (*E*). Postoperative maxillomandibular fixation to prevent excess tongue movement and flap dislodgement (*F*).

from the bilateral ventral surfaces. Laterally based ventral tongue flaps can be extended as far posteriorly as the circumvallate papilla and should not include any keratinized dorsal tongue mucosa to prevent the transfer of filliform and fungiform papilla. No floor of mouth mucosa should be included in the flap to prevent postoperative restriction in tongue mobility. The midline portion of the ventral tongue flap should not extend more posteriorly than 3 mm anterior to the submandibular caruncles to prevent injury to the submandibular ducts. At minimum, a thin cuff of muscle should be included with the flap to prevent vascular compromise, but the muscular bulk depends on the defect thickness. Undermining the tongue mucosa approximately 1 cm at the periphery of the flap incision aids in flap mobility.[19] The tongue tip can be sutured to the lower lip with a large silk tongue-lip adhesion suture to prevent dislodgement during the postoperative healing period. Appliances applied to the dentition are not necessary to prevent trauma to the flap. The tip of the tongue interpositioned between the teeth with the flap is sensate and prevents significant trauma.[17] The donor site of the ventral tongue can be closed primarily without significant morbidity. Second-stage surgery for flap division can occur any time between 14 and 21 days. The exposed tongue should be adequately moisturized from the time of inset and for 2 months postoperatively to prevent desiccation and chapping.[17,19]

Double- and Single-Door Tongue Flaps

Double- and single-door tongue flaps are horizontal, laterally based tongue flaps that are useful for lining large buccal mucosa and lingual alveolar defects. The flap can be extended from the midline of the tongue to the circumvallate papilla, allowing for reconstruction of defects extending from the commissures to the anterior ascending ramus. The flaps are raised by making an incision the length of the defect along the lateral border of the tongue. Superior and/or inferior flaps of approximately 5 to 7 mm in thickness are raised and rotated either superiorly or inferiorly and sutured to the margins of the defect. The flaps are left in place for 14 to 21 days postoperatively, and then second-stage surgery is performed for flap division. The defects of the tongue can be closed primarily at the time of second-stage surgery (**Fig. 5**). If a double-door flap is used, the 2 flaps are sutured together at the time of second-stage surgery for complete coverage of the defect. If the flaps are extended to reconstruct a buccal mucosal defect and patients are dentate, it is recommended that a bite

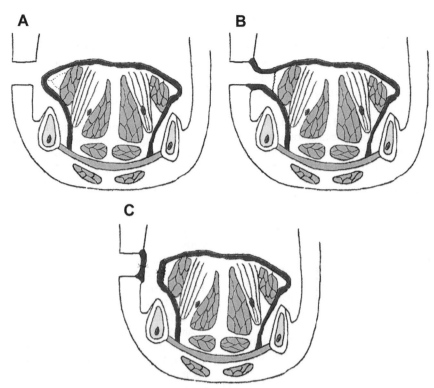

Fig. 5. Right buccal mucosa defect and outline of incision for double-door tongue flap (*A*). Double-door tongue flap inset into the buccal mucosa defect (*B*). Sectioned double-door tongue flap with complete reconstruction of the buccal mucosa defect (*C*).

block be inserted postoperatively to prevent trauma to the flaps.[1]

Lateral Tongue Flap

The lateral tongue flap is a robust flap that can be used for reconstruction of palatal, alveolar, buccal mucosal, retromolar trigone, lip, vermillion, commissure, and floor of mouth defects. The lateral tongue flap can be based anterior or posterior. Posteriorly based tongue flaps should not extend beyond the circumvallate papilla to prevent vascular compromise. Anterior-based lateral tongue flaps can extend to the midline. Creating a V-shaped wedge between the dorsal and ventral incisions aids in primary closure of the lateral tongue donor site defect.[11] The flap should include a cuff of muscle attached to the mucosa to prevent vascular compromise. No more than half of either hemitongue should be included in the flap to prevent significant postoperative functional deficits. Excessive rotation of the flap pedicle during inset can cause vascular compromise. The lateral tongue flap can be divided at 14 to 21 days. If the tongue flap traverses a dentate segment, a bite block may be indicated postoperatively to protect the flap pedicle.

Sliding and Island Tongue Flaps

Sliding and island tongue flaps can be used to reconstruct anterior, middle, and posterior tongue defects that are approximately 4 to 6 cm in size.[4,25] These moderate to large tongue defects cause significant functional problems if closed primarily or left to heal by secondary intent. Posterior tongue defects can be reconstructed using an anterior-based sliding tongue flap. The anterior-based sliding tongue flap is raised after division of the median fibrous septum to the anterior third of the tongue. The median fibrous septum is avascular, allowing for easy separation with minimal hemorrhage.[4,27] This division is carried through the genioglossus muscle and allows the tongue to be split into halves. The anterior extent of the incision is extended in a curvilinear fashion into the anterior third of the contralateral tongue. This contralateral extension allows for mobilization of the anterior-based sliding tongue flap that is then rotated posteriorly and inset into the posterior tongue defect and closed in a layered fashion. This rotation and advancement allow for primary closure of the defect and the incision line.[4] Similarly, anterior and middle tongue defects can be reconstructed with a posterior-based sliding tongue flap. Dissection begins with division of the median fibrous septum to the base of the tongue/vallecula. The suprahyoid musculature is then incised laterally, inferiorly, and posteriorly to allow for mobilization of the flap. Care must be taken to preserve the dorsal lingual artery. The posterior-based sliding tongue flap is then advanced into the anterior tongue defect and inset with a layered closure.[24] The tongue base island tongue flap is similar to the posterior-based sliding tongue flap in that it is based on the dorsal lingual artery and is used to reconstruct middle and anterior tongue defects. The tongue base island tongue flap allows for transfer of an appropriate-sized myomucosal paddle based on a small pedicle containing the dorsal lingual artery, instead of advancing the entire posterior hemitongue. This technique allows for a posterior-based flap that is less bulky and has increased mobility. This flap is more tenuous to prepare, because it requires careful dissection of the dorsal lingual artery. The tongue base island flap should be shaped approximately 1 cm smaller in size than the defect to allow for less tongue distortion. The donor defect can be closed primarily.[23]

Median Transit Tongue Flap

The median transit tongue flap is used to reconstruct anterior floor of the mouth defects. The median transit tongue flap is an anterior-based tongue flap that is created by elevating a 5- to 10-mm thick paddle from the contralateral dorsal tongue of appropriate size for the defect. Secondly, an incision of equal length to the width of the proposed flap is made through-and-through the median fibrous septum of the anterior tongue. This midline incision allows for a tunnel to be created through the anterior tongue. The flap is then tunneled through the median incision and inset into the contralateral anterior floor of the mouth defect.[27] The flap can be sectioned from days 14 to 21 to prevent tethering of the anterior tongue to the floor of the mouth.

COMPLICATIONS

The hardy nature of the tongue flap and its pliability and short length minimize some of the typical complications associated with other flaps, and a review of the literature revealed few articles describing such events. Most of the complications are temporary and minor and are associated with any surgery on the tongue. These include pain, swelling, bleeding, infection, hematoma, and temporary loss of tongue sensation. The only significant potential complications are speech issues, donor site deformity, premature flap detachment, and necrosis of the flap, and these are likely related to poor technique rather than intrinsic failure of flap.

Although it would seem that the inevitable alteration in the tongue's contour would lead to significant speech impediment, this does not seem to be the case as long as the mobility of the tip of the tongue is maintained.[45] Some donor site deformity can and does occur, regardless of whether or not the flap stump is returned to the tongue at takedown. This generally recontours itself with time to an acceptable level, but deferred recontouring can be performed at any time by scalpel, radiofrequency surgery, or laser (electrosurgical devices are best avoided due to muscle excitement and movement). Some narrowing of the tongue is expected, especially if the flap is not inset back into the tongue at takedown.[46]

Premature detachment of the flap from the defect site, although not common, is one of the more recognized and problematic complication.[47]

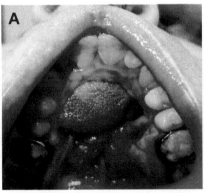 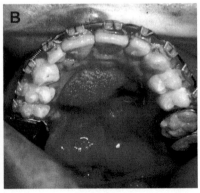

Fig. 6. Cleft palate patient with oronasal fistula previously reconstructed with a dorsal tongue flap. Bilateral oronasal fistulas recurred after Le Fort I osteotomy with advancement (*A*). Local tissue rearrangement used for closure (*B*).

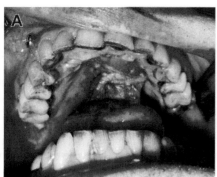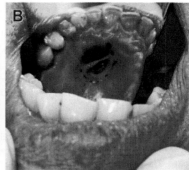

Fig. 7. Necrotic dorsal tongue flap secondary to excessive suture placement in the flap pedicle causing vascular compromise (*A*). Residual palatal defect after tongue flap failure (*B*).

This is caused by either excessive movement of the tongue in the postoperative period or inadequately securing the flap at the time of inset. Several techniques have been used to restrict tongue motion after surgery, including Kirschner wire fixation, stabilization of the tongue to the upper lip or incisors, placement of a Barton bandage or Jaw Bra, and maxillomandibular fixation.[32,46,48] When properly securing the flap and with the use of a soft mechanical or liquid diet, however, these seem unnecessary in most adult cases.[33,34] Small children may require some additional stabilization and also some mechanism to keep their fingers out of their mouths after surgery.

Some technical suggestions have been made in the literature in an attempt to prevent premature detachment. In 1976, Golden and colleagues[49] recommended the creation of an "aluminum suspension basket" (fashioned from the aluminum nasal splints commonly used at that time) wired to the teeth. More recently, Elyassi and colleagues[50] reported a "parachuting and anchoring" technique for oronasal fistulas that brought the flap up into the nose, allowing fixation not only in the palate but also in the nose itself for dual-level security. Once detachment has occurred, usually between 4 and 6 days postoperatively, reattachment is difficult due to the formation of granulation tissue and swelling of the flap. In 1995, Agrawal and Panda[51] reported a successful technique for reattachment using a silicone stent.

Like detachment, partial or complete necrosis of the flap is uncommon but can and does occur (**Fig. 6**). Given the robust nature of the flap and the supple blood supply, this complication is almost always a function of poor flap design. Inadequate length of the flap requiring tension during closure, overzealous rotation, and kinking of the flap and infection can all contribute to flap failure. When insetting the flap into the defect, there is great temptation to suture the muscle underlying the flap into the distal end of the defect. This must be avoided because the suture can interfere with the blood supply and strangulate the flap (**Fig. 7**). Partial necrosis can be managed with débridement, antibiotics, and wound irrigation. Complete necrosis requires débridement and reoperation.

SUMMARY

Although limited to anatomic defects located within a short arc of rotation, the dorsal or lateral tongue flap, when indicated, is a safe, reliable, and low-morbidity reconstructive option. It is particularly useful for defects in the palate, floor of mouth, pharynx, and buccal mucosa. Complications are rare and usually minor. It is imperative, however, that a well thought out strategy for airway management is planned, especially for the second-stage procedure.

REFERENCES

1. Domarus HV. The double-door tongue flap for total cheek mucosa defects. Plast Reconstr Surg 1988; 80:351–6.
2. Lexer E. Wangenplastik. Disch Z Chir 1909;100: 206.
3. Klopp CT, Schurter M. The surgical treatment of cancer of the soft palate and tonsil. Cancer 1956; 9:1239–43.
4. Lam DK, Cheng A, Berty KE, et al. Sliding anterior hemitongue flap for posterior tongue defect reconstruction. J Oral Maxillofac Surg 2012;70:2440–4.
5. Norton N. Netter's head and neck anatomy for dentistry. Philadelphia: Elsevier/Saunders; 2011.
6. Janfaza P, Nadol J, Galla R, et al. Surgical anatomy of the head and neck. Cambridge (MA): Harvard University Press; 2011.
7. Guzel MZ, Altintas F. Repair of large, anterior palatal fistulas using thin tongue flaps: long-term

follow-up of 10 patients. Ann Plast Surg 2000;45: 109–14.

8. Smith TS, Schaberg SJ, Collins JC. Repair of palatal defect using a dorsal pedicle tongue flap. J Oral Maxillofac Surg 1982;40:670–3.

9. Kim MJ, Lee JH, Choi JY, et al. Two-stage reconstruction of bilateral alveolar cleft using Y-shaped anterior-based tongue flap and iliac bone graft. Cleft Palate Craniofac J 2001;38:432–7.

10. Morel M, Danino A, Malka G. Use of the lateral tongue flap for closure of cleft palate. Retrospective study of seven cases. Ann Chir Plast Esthet 2001;46:5–9.

11. Sielgel EB, Bechtold W, Sherman PM, et al. Pedicle tongue flap for closure of an oroantral defect after partial maxillectomy. J Oral Surg 1977;35:746–9.

12. Minovi A, Ural A, Kollert M, et al. Lower lip reconstruction with the tongue flap: surgical technique and long-term results. B-ENT 2007;3:73–8.

13. Yuen JC, Zhou A, Shewmake K. Staged sequential reconstruction of a total lower lip, chin, and anterior mandible defect. Ann Plast Surg 1998;40: 297–301.

14. Hitoshi O, Koichi M, Yoshiyuki T, et al. A case of lower lip defect reconstructed with buccal mucosa and a tongue flap. J Craniofac Surg 2004; 15:614–7.

15. Yano K, Hosokawa K, Kubo T. Combined tongue flap and V-Y advancement flap for lower lip defects. Br J Plast Surg 2005;58:258–62.

16. Keskin M, Sutcu M, Tosun Z, et al. Reconstruction of total lower lip defects using radial forearm free flap with subsequent tongue flap. J Craniofac Surg 2010;21:349–51.

17. Doneland MB. Reconstruction of electrical burns of the oral commissure with a ventral tongue flap. Plast Reconstr Surg 1995;95:1155–63.

18. Guerrerosantos J, Trabanino C. Lower lip reconstruction with tongue flap in paramedian bilateral congenital sinuses. Plast Reconstr Surg 2002; 109:236–9.

19. Kheradmand AA, Garajei A. Ventral tongue myomucosal flap: a suitable choice for shaved lower vermillion border reconstruction. J Craniofac Surg 2013;24:e114–6.

20. Rees TD, Tabbal N, Aston SJ. Tongue-flap reconstruction of the lip vermillion in hemifacial atrophy. Plast Reconstr Surg 1983;72:643–7.

21. Cunha-Gomes D, Joshi PP, Bhathena H, et al. The lateral tongue flap: a salvage option for reconstruction of buccal recurrences. Acta Chir Plast 1999; 41:7–10.

22. Mehotra D, Pradhan R, Gupta S. Retrospective comparison of surgical treatment modalities in 100 patients with oral submucous fibrosis. Oral Surg Oral Med Oral Pathol Oral Radiol Endod 2009;107:e1–10.

23. Ye W, Hu J, Zhu H, et al. Tongue reconstruction with tongue base island advancement flap. J Craniofac Surg 2013;24:996–8.

24. Chicarilli ZN. Sliding posterior tongue flap. Plast Reconstr Surg 1987;79:687–700.

25. Schecter GL, Sly DE, Roper AL. Set back tongue flap for carcinoma of the tongue base. Arch Otolaryngol 1980;106:668–71.

26. Fischinger J, Zargi M. Repair of anterior floor of mouth defects by a central or paramedian island tongue flap. J Laryngol Otol 2003;117:391–5.

27. Calamel PM. The median transit tongue flap. Plast Reconstr Surg 1973;51:315–8.

28. Ceran C, Demirseren M, Sarici M, et al. Tongue flaps as a reconstructive option in intraoral defects. J Craniofac Surg 2013;24:972–4.

29. Lore JM, Klotch DW, Lee KY. One-staged reconstruction of the hypopharynx using myomucosal tongue flap and dermal graft. Am J Surg 1982; 144:473–6.

30. Zhang Q, Xing J, Song X, et al. The clinical study of tongue flaps repairing after resecting pharyngeal neoplasm and laryngeal neoplasm. Zhonghua Er Bi Yan Hou Ke Za Zhi 2000;35:371–3.

31. Sculerati N, Gottlieb MD, Zimbler MS, et al. Airway management in children with major craniofacial anomalies. Laryngoscope 1998;108:1806–12.

32. Kim YK, Yeo HH, Kim S. Use of the tongue flap for intraoral reconstruction: a report of 16 cases. J Oral Maxillofac Surg 1998;56:716–9.

33. Solan KJ. Nasal intubation and previous cleft palate repair. Anaesthesia 2004;59:923–4.

34. Hopkins JD, Jackson IT, Smith AW, et al. Large tongue flaps to close massive palatal defects. Eur J Plast Surg 1999;22:387–93.

35. Yamamoto K, Tsubokawa T, Ohmura S, et al. Left molar approach improves the laryngeal view in patients with difficult Laryngoscopy. Anesthesiology 2000;92:70–4.

36. Sahoo TK, Ambardekar M, Patel RD, et al. Airway management in a case of tongue flap division surgery: a case report. Indian J Anaesth 2009;53: 75–8.

37. Ying TS, Chin HN. Less traumatic method if inserting nasoendoctracheal tube in children. Paediatr Anaesth 2008;18:355–6.

38. Eipe N. Nasal intubation after tongue flap surgery. Acta Anesthesiol Scand 2009;53:269–74.

39. Peter S, Subash P, Paul J. Airway management during second-stage tongue flap procedure. Anesth Analg 2007;104:217.

40. Bracka A. The blood supply of dorsal tongue flaps for the closure of palatal fistulas. J Plast Surg 1981; 34:379–84.

41. Assuncao AG. The design of tongue flaps for the closure of palatal fistulas. Plast Reconstr Surg 1993;91:806–10.

42. Akinnebrew MC. Discussion, use of tongue flap for intraoral reconstruction: a case report of 16 cases. J Oral Maxillofac Surg 1998;56:720–1.
43. Deshmukh A, Kannan S, Thakkar P, et al. Tongue flap revisited. J Can Res Ther 2013;9:215–8.
44. Posnick JC, Getz SB. Surgical closure of end-stage palatal fistulas using anteriorly based dorsal tongue flaps. J Oral Maxillofac Surg 1987;45: 907–12.
45. Johnson PA, Banks P, Brown AA. The use of the posteriorly based lateral tongue flap in the repair of palatal fistule. Int J Oral Maxillofac Surg 1992; 21:6–9.
46. Zeidman A, Lockshin A, Berger J, et al. Repair of a chronic oronasal fistula defect with an anterior based tongue flap: report of a case. J Oral Maxillofac Surg 1988;46:412–5.
47. Guerrero-Santos J, Altimirano JT. The use of linguial flaps in the repair of fistulas of the hard palate. Plast Reconstr Surg 1996;38:123–8.
48. Fickling BW. Oral surgery involving the maxillary sinus. Ann R Coll Surg Engl 1957;20:537–42.
49. Golden GT, Mentzer RM, Fox JW, et al. "Basket suspension" as an adjust to tongue flap closure of hard palate defects. Cleft Palate J 1976;13: 350–3.
50. Elyassi AR, Helling ER, Closmann JJ. Closure of difficult palatal fistulas using a "parachuting and anchoring" technique with the tongue flap. Oral Surg Oral Med Oral Pathol Oral Radiol Endod 2011;1112:711–4.
51. Agrawal K, Panda KN. Management of a detached tongue flap. Plast Reconstr Surg 2007; 120:151–6.

Maxillofacial Reconstruction with Nasolabial and Facial Artery Musculomucosal Flaps

Daniel Cameron Braasch, DMD[a], Din Lam, DMD, MD[a],*,
Esther S. Oh, DDS, MD[b]

KEYWORDS

- Nasolabial • Facial artery musculomucosal flap • Facial artery • Maxillofacial reconstruction
- Intraoral defect

KEY POINTS

- The nasolabial flap is a random or axial patterned flap that can be used to reconstruct small to medium-sized perioral and intraoral defects up to 5×5 cm.
- The nasolabial flap is excellent for nasal tip reconstruction.
- The facial artery musculomucosal flap is an axial patterned flap used to provide vascularized mucosal tissue to defects of the oral cavity.
- Both flaps provide predictable results, with low morbidity.

INTRODUCTION

Resection of benign or malignant disease, traumatic injuries, and craniofacial abnormalities commonly result in maxillofacial defects requiring reconstruction. The ideal reconstructive technique should be focused on regaining both form and function. In perioral and intraoral reconstructive surgery, the importance of reestablishing function cannot be underestimated. The chosen technique should maintain or recreate oral competence, speech, deglutination and provide a cosmetic outcome. Ideally, the technique could be applied to multiple areas, have a low morbidity, and easy to incorporate into daily practice.

Local and systemic factors heavily influence the method of reconstruction. Locally, the size and site of the defect largely drive the method of reconstruction. Systemic factors must also be considered, including presence of diabetes, peripheral vascular disease, history of radiation or previous surgery, and most notably, previous neck dissection.

The nasolabial and facial artery musculomucosal (FAMM) flaps are pedicled flaps that provide versatility when reconstructing perioral and intraoral defects. These flaps provide soft tissue coverage for small to medium sized defects. The benefits of these flaps include the transfer of vascularized soft tissue, low harvest site morbidity, and ease of harvest.

NASOLABIAL FLAP

The nasolabial flap was first described by an Indian surgeon, Sushruta, in 700 BC.[1] The flap has gone through several modifications since its initial description. Nasolabial flaps have been applied to a variety of anatomic locations, such as the nose (lateral wall, ala and alar rim, tip), upper and lower lip, floor of mouth, tongue, palate, and alveolus.[2–4]

[a] Department of Oral and Facial Surgery, Virginia Commonwealth University Medical Center, 520 North 12th Street, Room 239, Richmond, VA 23298-0566, USA; [b] Department of Oral and Maxillofacial Surgery, University of Florida at Gainesville, 1395 Center Dr, Gainesville, FL 32603, USA
* Corresponding author.
E-mail address: dlam@vcu.edu

Oral Maxillofacial Surg Clin N Am 26 (2014) 327–333
http://dx.doi.org/10.1016/j.coms.2014.05.003
1042-3699/14/$ – see front matter © 2014 Elsevier Inc. All rights reserved.

The nasolabial flap has traditionally been described as an inferiorly based axial patterned flap based on the facial artery.[5] Anatomic studies have shown that in the nasolabial region, the arterial supply runs deep to the mimetic muscles (zygomaticus major and minor, levator anguli oris, nasalis, and quadrates oris). Throughout its course, the artery has vertically oriented perforator vessels, which run through the mimetic muscles to provide a rich blood supply to the subcutaneous tissue. The lower third of the nasolabial region has the most robust blood supply.[6] Only the nasolabial flaps that include the mimetic muscles and underlying artery should be considered true axial patterned flaps. Hynes and Boyd[7,8] showed that the blood supply in the subcutaneous tissue of the nasolabial region has an axial orientation. Based on these studies, the nasolabial flap can be harvested in the subcutaneous plane, but should be considered a random patterned flap.

The venous drainage in the nasolabial area is through the facial vein, which runs along the entire length of the region. It runs deep and lateral to the facial artery.

Indications and Contraindications

The nasolabial flap can be used to reconstruct small to medium-sized defects of the oral and maxillofacial region (**Table 1**). It is an ideal flap to reconstruct defects of the nose, because of its excellent color and texture match.[2] Furthermore, the flap can be used in conjunction with cartilaginous grafts to reconstruct defects of the ala.[9] Less commonly described, the flap has been used as a folded flap to reconstruct full-thickness defects, recreating both the skin and lining of the nose.[2,10] Although nasolabial flaps have been reported in the reconstruction of full nasal tip defects, the paramedian forehead flap is still preferred by most surgeons.[9]

The nasolabial flap is an excellent method to reconstruct defects of the upper lip. Unlike the Karapanzic and Abbe flaps, this flap does not result in microstomia and still reestablishes oral competence.[3,11,12] Even large full-thickness defects of the upper lip can be successfully reconstructed when the flap includes the underlying muscle. This flap provides an excellent cosmetic result, with significantly less morbidity and cost compared with free tissue transfer.[13]

For intraoral defects, the nasolabial flap can be tunneled through the buccal mucosa and inset in the floor of mouth, buccal mucosa, or palate.[4] This flap does not result in contracture and tissue tethering like other methods of reconstruction, such as skin grafts, especially when used in the floor of mouth and tongue. Free tissue transfer such as the radial forearm free flap can be used for floor of mouth or tongue reconstruction, but requires longer surgical time and specialized training in microvascular surgery. A major advantage of the nasolabial flap in floor of mouth reconstruction is excellent return to function. Hofstra and colleagues[13] reported minor effects on speech and the ability to wear a prosthesis, and only moderate effects on consumption of solid foods. This flap is best suited for small defect; however, reconstruction of larger defects has also been reported with bilateral nasolabial flaps.

There are few contraindications to the nasolabial flap. Relative contraindications include previous neck dissection, simultaneous free flap surgery using the facial artery, history of radiation, defects greater than 5 cm × 5 cm, and sites distant to the arc of rotation.

Surgical Procedure

Preoperative planning and preparation
The nasolabial flap requires minimal preoperative planning. The skin laxity in the midface should be evaluated, because increased laxity in this region allows for easy tension-free closure of the harvest site and a more cosmetic result. When designing the flap, it should contain skin outside hair-bearing regions to prevent transfer of hair to intraoral sites. If hair growth does occur at the recipient site, secondary hair removal procedures may be required.

The recipient site should be completely prepared before flap harvesting to ensure that enough tissue can be obtained from unilateral or bilateral nasolabial flaps. Furthermore, the arc of rotation must be evaluated to ensure that the flap can be rotated to the recipient site without significant tension.

Reconstruction of extraoral defects, such as on the nose or lips, can be completed under local anesthesia, intravenous sedation, or general anesthesia. The oral cavity should be kept out of the field to prevent contamination. If planning intraoral defect reconstruction, general anesthesia with nasoendotracheal tube intubation is preferred. A

Table 1	
Indications for nasolabial and FAMM flaps	
Indications for Nasolabial Flap	**Indications for FAMM Flap**
Superior based flap	Superior based flap
Nose (lateral wall, tip, ala)	Palate
	Nasal septum
Inferior based flap	Upper lip
Upper lip	Inferior based flap
Buccal mucosa	Floor of mouth
Floor of mouth	Lower lip
Palate	Tongue
	Gingival alveolus

throat pack should be used, and the intraoral and extraoral sites should be prepared and scrubbed with chlorhexidine or betadine.

Inferiorly based flap

For full-thickness axial patterned flaps, doppler is helpful to trace the course of the facial and angular arteries to ensure that the flap is centered over the arterial supply. Gauze can then be used to evaluate the arc of rotation to the defect site, with minimal tension and twisting. The superior aspect can be extended superiorly to about 0.5 to 0.75 cm medial or anterior to the medial canthus.[14] If the flap harvest is carried too close to the medial canthus, then, primary closure may not be possible. The base of the flap can extend inferiorly to the level of the oral commissure. Flaps extending to the inferior border of the mandible have been reported, but are not routinely used.[15] The medial aspect of the flap is 1 to 2 mm lateral to the nasolabial fold. If the incision is located within the fold, a flattened appearance results when the harvest site is primarily closed, which appears asymmetric and unaesthetic.

The nasolabial flap can be designed as a 1-staged or 2-staged flap. Single-staged flaps are ideal for reconstruction of perioral defects, some nasal defects, and buccal mucosa defects. Reconstruction of the floor of mouth and tongue requires a 2-stage procedure.[16] The second stage should be delayed for 3 to 4 weeks.

Surgical Procedure

The planned incision line is injected with local anesthesia with vasoconstrictor 5 minutes before incision to provide a dry field of dissection. The flap is raised from superior to inferior and from medial to lateral. If a full-thickness flap is planned, dissection is carried through the mimetic muscles, and the facial or angular artery is identified and raised with the flap. Doppler helps ensure that the artery remains in the flap throughout the harvest.

For random-pattern flaps, dissection begins at the distal end of the flap and carried in the subcutaneous plane but above the muscular layer. When used for extraoral reconstruction, the flap is rotated to the recipient site and sutured into place (**Fig. 1**). During

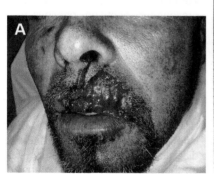
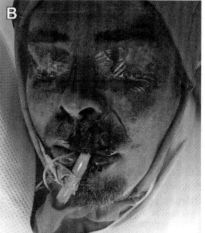
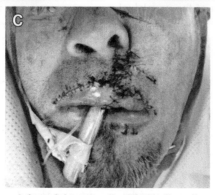

Fig. 1. (*A*) Traumatic partial-thickness defect of the upper lip. (*B*) The dimension of nasolabial flap is outlined in red; Black arrows demonstrate the rotation of the flap. A separated vermillion advancement flap is raised to cover the vermillion defect. (*C*) Immediate postoperative result showing closure of a traumatic defect with a single-stage nasolabial flap.

intraoral reconstruction, the inferior 1.5 to 2 cm must be de-epithelialized to allow passage into the oral cavity. A transbuccal tunnel of 1.5 to 2 cm is created to allow easy passage to the oral cavity.

The donor site must be closed primarily in a tension-free fashion. The tissue lateral to the harvest site is aggressively undermined in a supramuscular plane to prevent damage to the facial nerve. Lack of adequate dissection results in closure under tension, which may lead to incision line breakdown or scar formation.

For two-stage procedure, flap needs to be revised and divided 3 weeks to 4 weeks after the initial surgery. During its second stage, flap should be appropriately thinned and contoured. The intervening tissue can either be inset in the receipt site if additional tissue is required or discarded.

Complications

The nasolabial flap is a predictable method of reconstruction. The most common minor complications include partial flap necrosis, usually at the distal aspect of the flap, and flap dehiscence. These complications are easily managed with local debridement and reclosure. Rare complications include complete flap necrosis, orocutaneous fistula, inclusion cyst, oral incompetence, and speech difficulty.

Current Controversies/Future Considerations

The most controversial topic with nasolabial flaps is its use in patients with previous neck dissections. Originally, the flap was believed to be a true axial patterned flap, based on the facial and angular arteries. During a neck dissection, the facial artery is often ligated, which results in disruption of blood flow to the nasolabial region. The flap is rarely harvested as an axial patterned flap in this case. Instead, it is raised with a random patterned blood supply. Several studies[4,5,14,16–19] have shown the successful use of the nasolabial flap in combination with ipsilateral neck dissection. The ability to use a nasolabial flap despite ipsilateral neck dissection is a result of the extensive blood supply to the region.

The use of radiation has also been suggested as a contraindication for the use of the flap. However, several studies[13,20] have shown the successful use of this flap in radiated patients with no increased risk of complications.

THE FAMM FLAP

The facial artery musculomucosal flap was originally described by Dr Julian Pribaz[21] in 1992 for the correction of oronasal mucosal defects. This intraoral flap is an axial patterned flap, based on the facial artery. The facial artery branches off the external carotid artery and travels superiorly over the inferior border of the mandible. The artery has a diameter of 1.4 to 4.7 mm, with an average diameter of 2.6 mm as it crosses the inferior border of the mandible.[22,23] At the level of the oral commissure, the facial artery is located about 15.5 mm lateral to the commissure and gives off 3 to 5 branches before its termination. The termination of the facial artery is highly variable, **Fig. 2**B shows 1 of 5 possible paths.[23] The artery runs deep to the risorius and zygomaticus, but superficial to the buccinators, levator anguli oris, and obicularis oris muscles.[24] Because of the robust blood supply from the facial artery, the flap can be designed with either an inferior based and rely on antegrade blood flow or a superior based with retrograde blood flow.[21] When harvesting the flap, the mucosa, submucosa, buccinator, and obicularis oris are incorporated into the flap.

Indications/Contraindications

The FAMM flap has been successfully used for the reconstruction of defects of the palate, nasal septum, skull base, floor of mouth, upper and lower lip, tongue, and alveolus (see **Table 1**).[21,25–28] Relative contraindications include presence of dentition, previous neck dissection, and history of radiation. Lack of a doppler signal along the path of the facial artery is an absolute contraindication to using this flap.

Surgical Procedure

Preoperative planning

Unlike free tissue transfer, the FAMM flap requires little preoperative workup. The most important diagnostic workup is to establish a doppler signal on the facial artery before entering the operating room. This step is necessary to ensure a fully functional facial artery, especially when the patient has undergone ipsilateral neck dissection or radiation treatment to the head and neck. Anatomical studies have shown variability in the facial artery, with the potential for a hypoplastic or rudimentary facial artery that terminates before the commissure. Lack of a fully developed facial artery prevents the harvest of a FAMM flap.[29]

Preparation

Nasotracheal intubation generally recommended for oral cavity reconstruction. The path of the facial artery is traced from the facial notch extraorally to its termination lateral to the ala of the nose. Intraorally, doppler is also used to trace the path from the retromolar pad to its superior extent in the

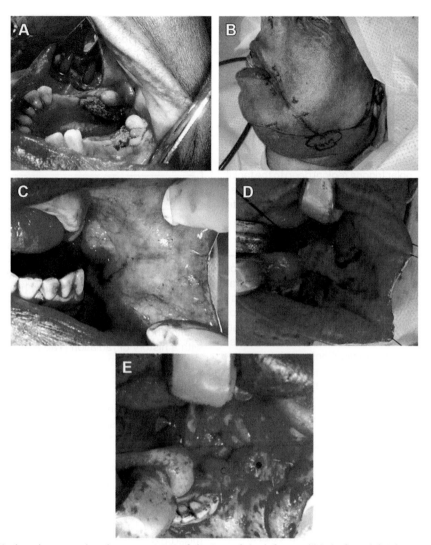

Fig. 2. (*A*) Bisphosphonate-related osteonecrosis of the jaw of the left mandible before debridement. (*B*) Extraoral mapping of the facial artery. ILA, inferior labial artery; SLA, superior labial artery. (*C*) Intraoral mapping of the facial artery. (*D*) Mobilization of the FAMM flap. (*E*) Immediate postoperative photograph showing inset of the FAMM flap and closure of the donor site with Alloderm® (LifeCell Corporation, Branchburg, NJ). Black circle, donor site; blue circle, recipient site.

gingivobuccal sulcus (see **Fig. 2**A–C). To aid in dissection of the flap, 2 sutures can be placed superior and inferior to the commissure to create a taut buccal mucosa (see **Fig. 2**D).

Inferiorly based flap

After the path of the facial artery is determined, the flap is outlined. The first incision is traditionally made either at the distal extent of the flap or at the level of the oral commissure. With the aid of doppler, sharp dissection is used to dissect through the buccinator muscle to identify the facial artery. At the distal extent of the flap, the facial artery is ligated. Dissection is then carried from distal to proximal direction. Care should be made to incorporate small cuff of buccinators muscle to protect the facial artery (see **Fig. 2**D). The flap can be up to 2 to 3 cm wide, but care must be taken to ensure that dissection is anterior to the Stenson duct.

When the flap has been fully mobilized, one can either rotate the tissue to the defect or create a submucosal tunnel to the recipient site (see **Fig. 2**E). When transferring the flap to the recipient site, care should be taken to prevent twisting of the pedicle, which could result in kinking of the facial artery and disrupting its blood supply. Once the flap is inset into the recipient site, doppler can be used to confirm that the facial artery has not been kinked. The donor site can be closed primarily with a 2-layer closure: muscle and then mucosa. Alternatively, the harvest site can be covered with AlloDerm® Regenerative Tissue Matrix (LifeCell Corporation, Branchburg, NJ) or skin graft if primary closure cannot be obtained.

Superiorly based flap

A superiorly based flap relies on retrograde blood flow through the facial artery. The preoperative preparation is the same as an inferiorly based flap, with confirmation of the arterial supply using doppler. The flap is harvested from its distal end (near the retromolar trigone region) deep to the facial artery. After the flap is fully mobilized, it can be transferred to the recipient site. Closure of the harvest site is carried out the same as an inferiorly based flap.

Complications

Complications of the FAMM flap include partial or complete flap necrosis, dehiscence, hematoma, infection, and speech difficulty. If flap necrosis occurs, it is likely to be at the most distal aspect of the flap.[30–32] Partial necrosis and dehiscence can be managed by local debridement and reclosure. Prevention of most complications can be accomplished by ensuring that the arterial supply remains in the flap during harvest and that there is no kinking of the artery during inset. When FAMM flap is used to reconstruct an oral-nasal fistula, recurrence is uncommon. Failure in fistula closure is most likely due to heavy scar tissue from the previous surgery.[31]

Current Controversies

Currently, the biggest debate concerns the FAMM flap in patients who have undergone previous neck dissection or radiation. Ligation of the facial artery during neck dissection theoretically precludes the use of the FAMM flap. Preliminary studies have shown the successful use of the FAMM flap in all but 2 patients with ipsilateral and bilateral neck dissections (**Table 2**).

Table 2
Previous neck dissection and FAMM flap success rate

Study	Number of Patients	Partial Necrosis	Complete Necrosis
Bianchi et al,[30] 2009	22	1	1
Ayad et al,[32] 2008	39	Unknown	0
O'Leary et al,[33] 2011	14	Unknown	0
Parrett et al,[34] 2012	4	0	0

Table 3
Radiation and FAMM flap successful rate

Study	Number of Patients	Partial Necrosis	Complete Necrosis
Ayad et al,[32] 2008	10	Unknown	0
O'Leary & Bundgaard,[33] 2011	4	1	0
Parrett et al,[34] 2012	3	0	0

Although a side effect of radiation could result in decreased blood flow through the facial artery, 3 studies[32–34] with a total of 17 patients have used the FAMM flap in patients with a history of radiation. None resulted in complete necrosis of the flap, and only 1 patient had partial necrosis, indicating the potential use of the flap in patients with a history of radiation (**Table 3**).

SUMMARY

The nasolabial and FAMM flaps are predictable methods to reconstruct perioral and intraoral defects with vascularized tissue. The nasolabial flap can be harvested as an axial or random patterned flap, whereas the FAMM flap is truly an axial patterned flap, with either a superiorly or inferiorly based. Both flaps have been widely used to provide predictable results, with low morbidity. Future studies are needed to further prove their use in compromised patients, including patients with a history of head and neck radiation and neck dissections.

REFERENCES

1. Pers M. Cheek flaps in partial rhinoplasty. Scand J Plast Reconstr Surg 1967;1:37–42.
2. Turan A, Kul Z, Turkaslan T, et al. Reconstruction of lower half defects of the nose with the lateral nasal artery pedicle nasolabial island flap. Plast Reconstr Surg 2007;119(6):1767–72.
3. Tan NC, Hsieh CH, Riva FM, et al. The nasolabial flap as a one-stage procedure for reconstruction of intermediate-to-large lip defects with functional and aesthetic assessments. J Plast Reconstr Aesthet Surg 2013;66(3):352–7.
4. Varghese BT, Sebastian P, Cherian T, et al. Nasolabial flaps in oral reconstruction: an analysis of 224 cases. Br J Plast Surg 2001;54(6):499–503.
5. Birt BD, Gruss JS. Intra-oral reconstruction using the nasolabial flap. J Otolaryngol 1985;14(4):233–6.

6. Hagan WE, Walker LB. The nasolabial musculocutaneous flap: clinical and anatomical correlations. Laryngoscope 1988;98(3):341–6.

7. Hynes B, Boyd JB. The nasolabial flap. Axial or random? Arch Otolaryngol Head Neck Surg 1988; 114(12):1389–91.

8. Drake RL, Vogl WA, Mitchell AWM. Head and neck. In: Livingstone C, editor. Gray's anatomy for students. 2nd edition. Philadelphia: Elsevier; 2010. p. 856–72.

9. Paddack AC, Frank RW, Spencer HJ, et al. Outcomes of paramedian forehead and nasolabial interpolation flaps in nasal reconstruction. Arch Otolaryngol Head Neck Surg 2012;138(4):367–71.

10. Kearney C, Sheridan A, Vinciullo C, et al. A tunneled and turned-over nasolabial flap for reconstruction of full thickness nasal ala defects. Dermatol Surg 2010; 36(8):1319–24.

11. Rudkin GH, Carlsen BT, Miller TA. Nasolabial flap reconstruction of large defects of the lower lip. Plast Reconstr Surg 2003;111(2):810–7.

12. Cook JL. The reconstruction of two large full-thickness wounds of the upper lip with different operative techniques: when possible, a local flap repair is preferable to reconstruction with free tissue transfer. Dermatol Surg 2013;39(2):281–9.

13. Hofstra EI, Hofer SO, Nauta JM, et al. Oral functional outcome after intraoral reconstruction with nasolabial flaps. Br J Plast Surg 2004;57(2):150–5.

14. Ducic Y, Burye M. Nasolabial flap reconstruction of oral cavity defects: a report of 18 cases. J Oral Maxillofac Surg 2000;58(10):1104–8.

15. Borle RM, Nimonkar PV, Rajan R. Extended nasolabial flaps in the management of oral submucous fibrosis. Br J Oral Maxillofac Surg 2009;47(5):382–5.

16. Lazaridis N, Tilaveridis I, Karakasis D. Superiorly or inferiorly based "islanded" nasolabial flap for buccal mucosa defects reconstruction. J Oral Maxillofac Surg 2008;66(1):7–15.

17. Lazaridis N. Unilateral subcutaneous pedicled nasolabial island flap for anterior mouth floor reconstruction. J Oral Maxillofac Surg 2003;61(2):182–90.

18. Napolitano M, Mast BA. The nasolabial flap revisited as an adjunct to floor-of-mouth reconstruction. Ann Plast Surg 2001;46(3):265–8.

19. El Khatib K, Danino A, Trost O, et al. Use of nasolabial flap for mouth floor reconstruction. Ann Chir Plast Esthet 2005;50(3):216–20.

20. Maurer P, Eckert AW, Schubert J. Functional rehabilitation following resection of the floor of the mouth: the nasolabial flap revisited. J Craniomaxillofac Surg 2002;30(6):369–72.

21. Pribaz J, Stephens W, Crespo L, et al. A new intraoral flap: facial artery musculomucosal (FAMM) flap. Plast Reconstr Surg 1992;90(3):421–9.

22. Jiang GH, Yan JH, Lin CL, et al. Anatomic study of the facial artery using multislice spiral CT angiography. Nan Fang Yi Ke Da Xue Xue Bao 2008; 28(3):457–9 [in Chinese].

23. Pinar YA, Bilge O, Govsa F. Anatomic study of the blood supply of perioral region. Clin Anat 2005; 18(5):330–9.

24. Niranjan NS. An anatomical study of the facial artery. Ann Plast Surg 1988;21(1):14–22.

25. Joshi A, Rajendraprasad JS, Shetty K. Reconstruction of intraoral defects using facial artery musculomucosal flap. Br J Plast Surg 2005;58(8):1061–6.

26. Pribaz JJ, Meara JG, Wright S, et al. Lip and vermilion reconstruction with the facial artery musculomucosal flap. Plast Reconstr Surg 2000;105(3): 864–72.

27. Heller JB, Gabbay JS, Trussler A, et al. Repair of large nasal septal perforations using facial artery musculomucosal (FAMM) flap. Ann Plast Surg 2005;55(5):456–9.

28. Xie L, Lavigne F, Rahal A, et al. Facial artery musculomucosal flap for reconstruction of skull base defects: a cadaveric study. Laryngoscope 2013; 123(8):1854–61.

29. Mitz V, Ricbourg B, Lassau JP. Facial branches of the facial artery in adults. Typology, variations and respective cutaneous areas. Ann Chir Plast 1973; 18(4):339–50.

30. Bianchi B, Ferri A, Ferrari S, et al. Myomucosal cheek flaps: applications in intraoral reconstruction using three different techniques. Oral Surg Oral Med Oral Pathol Oral Radiol Endod 2009;108(3): 353–9.

31. Lahiri A, Richard B. Superiorly based facial artery musculomucosal flap for large anterior palatal fistulae in clefts. Cleft Palate Craniofac 2007;44(5):523–7.

32. Ayad T, Kolb F, De Monés E, et al. Reconstruction of floor of mouth defects by the facial artery musculomucosal flap following cancer ablation. Head Neck 2008;30(4):437–45.

33. O'Leary P, Bundgaard T. Good results in patients with defects after intraoral tumour excision using facial artery musculo-mucosal flap. Dan Med Bull 2011;58(5):A4264.

34. Parrett BM, Przylecki WH, Singer MI. Reliability of the facial artery musculomucosal flap for intraoral reconstruction in patients who have undergone previous neck dissection and radiation therapy. Plast Reconstr Surg 2012;130(6):910e–2e.

Lip Reconstruction

 CrossMark

Mehdi B. Matin, DDS, Jasjit Dillon, DDS, MBBS, FDSRCS*

KEYWORDS

- Lip reconstruction • Partial-thickness defect • Full-thickness defect • Local and regional flap

KEY POINTS

- Small to moderate lip defects should be repaired with local and regional flaps.
- Local and regional flaps can provide both cosmetic and functional lip reconstruction.
- Microstomia is a common sequela in subtotal lip reconstruction.
- Microvascular reconstruction provides an excellent option for complex or total lip reconstruction; however, it lacks the ability of providing any dynamic function.

INTRODUCTION

The lips consist of 2 fleshy folds that surround the mouth in humans. They play a dynamic role in facial esthetics, human communications, and oral functions, such as producing sounds, facial expressions, and providing an oral seal.[1–3]

Defects may result from trauma, malignancy, and congenital disorders.[4] These defects may cause significant alterations of normal lip appearance and function that profoundly impact patients' quality of life.[5] Therefore presents significant challenges for a surgeon to restore form and function of this complex vital anatomic unit. Although lip attempts to restore all of the above, oral competence is probably the most important.[6]

Surgical management of patients in need of lip reconstruction requires a clear understanding of the lip anatomy, aesthetics, and function[7] as well as extensive knowledge and background information of various techniques proposed to this date. This article is a comprehensive review of lip defects reconstruction.

HISTORY

The first evidence of lip reconstruction is found as far back as the Hindu and Sanskrit writings of Sushruta. In 600 BC, Sushruta, an Indian surgeon,

published the first written description of lip reconstruction. Early reports of lip reconstruction in the Western literature date back to at least the first century.[1,8]

Many modern techniques are combinations and newer modification of methods first described by Dieffenbach, Sabatini, Abbe, and Estlander[9–14] over the past 2 centuries. In 1834, Dieffenbach[9,10] first described the cheek advancement flap technique based on an inferolateral pedicle. In 1838, Sabatini[11] first described the cross-lip flap transfer of the lower lip midline wedge to a philtral defect. This technique was modified and further popularized by Abbe and Estlander.[12,13] In 1853, Bernard[15] explained his technique of full-thickness wedge excision and cheek advancement for the repair of a lower lip defect. Earlier techniques, such as bilateral nasolabial flaps (von Bruns[16] 1857) and fan flap (Gillies[17] 1920s) using full-thickness flaps, led to denervation and did not allow for functional restoration.[18] Later Karapandzic[19] improved Gillies' technique with the preservation of underlying musculature and neurovascular structures. The utilization of microvascular free tissue transfer for total lip reconstruction was first reported by Harri and colleagues in 1974.[20,21] Later complex reconstructive options, such as functional gracilis transfer, were elaborated to meet the requirements of lip reconstruction[20]; and recently, successful

Disclosures: None.
Department of Oral & Maxillofacial Surgery, University of Washington, 1959 Northeast Pacific Street, HSB Room B 241, Box 357134, Seattle, WA 98195, USA
* Corresponding author.
E-mail address: dillonj5@uw.edu

partial facial transplantation makes this technique an increasingly more likely option for reconstruction in coming years.[20,22,23]

ANATOMIC CONSIDERATIONS

It is necessary to have an in-depth understanding of anatomy in order to achieve superior outcomes in lip reconstructive surgeries. Lips are located within the observation of the lower face, and even minor defects require meticulous reconstruction.[5] The normal lip considerably varies in width, length, and thickness among patients. The anatomic boundaries of the lips extend vertically from the subnasale to the chin and horizontally from commissure to commissure.[1,5,6,24]

Anatomic development of the lips begins in the early embryonic stage. The maxilla, mandible, and both lips are derived from the first pharyngeal arch. Upper lip development is from the fusion of maxillary and medial nasal prominences with the intermaxillary segment. The commissure is formed by fusion of the lateral portion of the maxillary and mandibular processes. Lower lip and mandible are derived from mandible process as a single structure.[3]

The *cross-sectional anatomy* (**Fig. 1**) of the lips, from superficial to deep, consists of skin (epidermis, dermis, subcutaneous tissue), orbicularis oris muscle fibers, and submucosal and mucosal layers. Lips are surrounded by skin externally and transition to internal mucosa at the mucocutaneous ridge or vermilion border, which is the most distinguishing feature of the lip.[1,24] A fine line of pale skin, *white roll*, accentuates the color difference between the vermilion and skin. The mucosa of the vermilion is unique in that it lacks minor salivary glands. The line separating this dry portion from intraoral labial mucosa is called the *wet line*. The characteristic hue of the vermilion comes from a rich underlying vascular supply and thin keratinized stratified squamous epithelium. This vascular bed and neural plexus makes the vermilion highly sensate.[25]

The upper lip consists of a middle and 2 lateral *aesthetic subunits* (**Figs. 2** and **3**), demarcated by the philtral ridges medially and the nasolabial folds laterally. The central concavity between vermilion and subnasale is called the *philtral groove*, which is limited bilaterally by philtral ridges.[3,5] The central depression of the upper vermilion is referred to as *cupid's bow*. The lower lip is composed of a single subunit considerably less complex and more forgiving to reconstruct. It is separated from the surrounding structures by a labiomental crease and melolabial fold. The labiomental

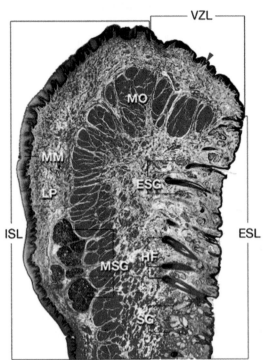

Fig. 1. Lip cross section. ESG, eccrine sweat; ESL, external side of lip; HF, hair follicles; ISL, internal side of lip; LP, lamina propria; MM, the mucous membrane (stratified squamous nonkeratinized epithelium); MO, muscularis orbicularis oris; MSG, minor salivary glands; SG, sebaceous glands (associated with hair follicles); VZL, vermillion (red) zone. (*From* Arda O, Göksügür N, Tüzün Y. Basic histological structure and functions of facial skin. Clin Dermatol 2014;32(1):3–13; with permission.)

crease forms an inverted *U*, which corresponds to the depth of gingivolabial sulcus.

Adequate *vascularization* is a critical element of flaps in reconstructive surgery.[4] Both lips receive their blood supply from the facial branch of the external carotid artery via the superior and inferior labial branches that course between the orbicularis oris muscle fibers and the mucosa and just deep to posterior vermilion line. According to Neligan,[25] the superior labial artery runs through the muscle in half of patients and has a tendency to travel slightly higher in the central parts of the upper lip. It anastomoses contralaterally and communicates with the subdermal plexus.[1,3] Venus drainage runs with the arteries but, in the upper lip, can drain to the cavernous sinus via the ophthalmic vein, providing a route for labial infections to spread intracranially.[3]

Lymphatic drainage of the lips merges to 5 primary trunks. The upper lip, except the midline, drains ipsilaterally to the submandibular nodes

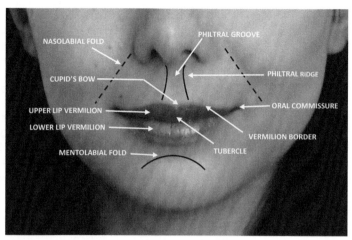

Fig. 2. Anatomic landmarks of lip.

with some drainage to the periparotid nodes and occasionally to the submental nodes. The lower lip drains bilaterally to the submental nodes in the center and submandibular nodes laterally.[26]

Sensation of the upper and lower lips is provided by the infraorbital branch of maxillary division and the mental branch of mandibular division of the trigeminal nerve, respectively.[3]

The *motor supply* is derived primarily from buccal and marginal mandibular branches of the facial nerve. These nerves enter deep into

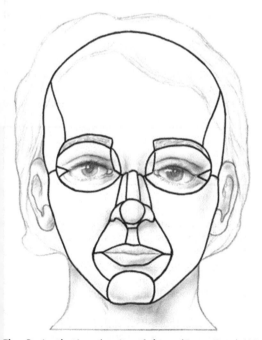

Fig. 3. Aesthetic subunits of face. (*From* Patel KG, Sykes JM. Concepts in local flap design and classification. Oper Tech Otolaryngol–Head Neck Surg 2011; 22(1):13–23; with permission.)

muscles, except the mentalis, which receives superficial innervation.[25–27]

Perioral musculature (**Fig. 4**) can be classified as 3 groups based on insertion into the commissure (modiolus) and upper and lower lip. **Table 1** shows the groups as well as the function of each muscle.[26] The orbicularis oris principally composes the body of the lip. Deep fibers provide the oral cavity sphincter function, whereas the superficial fibers perform fine movements.[27] In the cross section, the orbicularis oris is composed of a long, vertical segment that curls outward at the superior and inferior free margins to form a marginal protrusion. In the upper lip, the orbicularis oris fibers decussate in the midline and have dermal insertions approximately 4 to 5 mm lateral from the midline. This serves to pull the skin medially at these dermal insertion points, forming the philtral columns. The central region (philtral groove) is devoid of dermal attachments and is pulled into a concave depression.[26]

PATHOLOGY AND EPIDEMIOLOGY

Cancer resection causes most lip defects; however, trauma; burns; and certain disease processes, such as granulomatous cheilitis, hemangioma, nevi, melanotic macules, and noma, can cause lip defects that require reconstructive surgery. Unlike facial and lip skin where basal cell carcinoma (BCC) is the most common malignancy, squamous cell carcinoma (SCC) constitutes 95% of primary malignant lesions of the red lip followed by BCC, melanoma, minor salivary gland malignancies, microcystic adnexal carcinoma, and Merkel cell carcinoma.[3,28]

Lip cancer accounts for 25% of oral cavity malignancies, and its incidence can be as high as

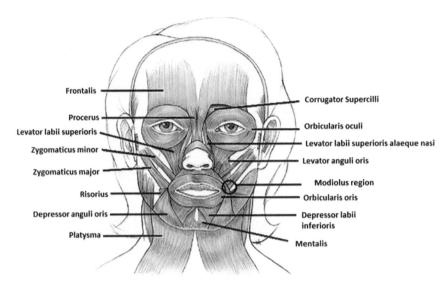

Fig. 4. Perioral musculature. (*Modified from* Gillman GS, Gallo JF. Cosmetic uses of Botox and injectable fillers. In: Bailey BJ, Johnson JT, Newlands SD, editors. Head & neck surgery–otolaryngology. 4th edition. Philadelphia: Lippincott Williams & Wilkins; 2006.)

13.5 per 100,000 people.[28] The risk factors for lip cancer include sun exposure, smoking, alcohol consumption, and fair complexion. It is 3 to 13 times more common in males.[3,28–30] Lower lips receive more ultraviolet exposure and are the most common site for lip cancers (89%); although rarer, carcinomas from upper lips (7%) and commissures (4%) are more aggressive.[3,28]

GENERAL CONSIDERATIONS

Management of lip defects with reconstructive surgery requires restoration of labial/oral function and restoration of esthetics. There are several options for defect reconstruction[24,25,31] and will vary per patient (**Box 1**).

FUNCTIONAL AND ESTHETIC CONSIDERATIONS

Box 2 lists some of the most important functional and aesthetic goals of reconstructive surgeries. Three-layered closure, reconstruction of orbicularis oris, and restoration of the continuity of the lips sphincter and labial vestibules are essential to restore ideal function. Microstomia is a common complication in lip reconstruction that could affect function. In order to avoid microstomia, bringing new tissue to the lip might be necessary.[1,3,6,27]

Topographic boundaries and aesthetic subunits (see **Figs. 2** and **3**) must be recognized and respected.[4] It is best to avoid crossing these

Table 1
Perioral musculature

Muscle Group	Muscle	Action
Group I: modiolus insertion	Orbicularis oris	Presses the lips against the teeth
	Buccinator	Presses the lips and cheek against the teeth
	Levator anguli oris	Elevates the commissure
	Depressor anguli oris	Depresses and moves the commissure laterally
	Zygomaticus major	Elevates and moves the commissure laterally
	Risorius	Draws the commissure laterally and smiling
Group II: upper lip insertion	Levator labii superioris	Elevates the upper lip
	Levator labii superioris alaeque nasi	Dilates the nostril and elevates the upper lip
	Zygomaticus minor	Elevates and pulls the commissure laterally
Group III: lower lip insertion	Depressor labii inferioris	Depresses the lower lip and pulls it slightly laterally
	Mentalis	Elevates the lower lip
	Platysma	Depresses the lips

Box 1
Patient and defect factors affecting treatment plan

- Patient factor
  - Age
  - Prognosis
  - General medical condition
  - Patient compliance
  - Comorbidities
  - Cost and convenience of treatment
- Defect/tumor factor
  - Size of tumor
  - Histology of tumor
  - Extent of lip resection/defect
  - Anticipation of esthetic and functional outcome
  - Availability of local tissue
  - History of prior treatment (eg, radiation and surgery)

Data from Refs.[24,28,32]

boundaries. When a defect involves a substantial portion of an esthetic subunit, better cosmetic results are achieved by reconstructing areas as complete units.[3]

Box 2
The most important reconstructive goals are outlined as follows

- Functional goal
  - Maintenance of oral competence
  - Sufficient oral access
  - Preservation of sensation
  - Mobility
  - Phonation
- Aesthetic goal
  - Restore or preservation of the anatomic land marks
  - Reconstruction of facial subunits
  - Adequate tissue match in terms of color and texture
  - Lip symmetry and anatomic proportion
  - Maintenance of lips relation

Data from Refs.[3,5,24,32,33]

RECONSTRUCTIVE STRATEGIES OF UPPER AND LOWER LIPS

Lip defects are classified based on anatomic location, thickness, and size of the defect (**Box 3**).[34] The main reconstructive options include secondary intention healing, skin grafts, primary closure, local flaps, and free flaps. When considering reconstruction of lip defect, the *reconstruction ladder* starts with the simplest procedures, moving up to the most complex.[32] **Figs. 5–7** show the basic approach to lip defects from simple to complex. This classification has limitations but helps to have an organized approach to this problem.

Vermilion Defects

The vermilion is the most distinguishing feature of the lip and consists of specialized stratified squamous epithelium.[34] The junction between the vermilion and white lip (white roll) is smooth and seamless; any abnormality is immediately obvious, which makes vermilion reconstruction critical.

Healing by secondary intention
Small, partial-thickness defects of the lip isolated to the vermilion or extending marginally to the cutaneous lip that do not involve the underlying orbicularis muscle may heal nicely through secondary intention.[3,35–38] Leonard and Hanke[39] reported re-epithelialization of such defects by 25 days on average, with good cosmetic results without persistent visible scar. Wound contraction is still a disadvantage and should be anticipated.[40]

Primary closure
For a small vermilion defect in which the remaining vermilion shape and contour is not distorted,

Box 3
Defect classification

- Anatomic location
  - Skin
  - Vermilion
  - Skin and vermilion
- Thickness
  - Partial thickness
  - Full thickness
- Size
  - Small less than 30% of lip
  - Medium 30% to 60% of lip width
  - Subtotal or total greater than 60% lip width

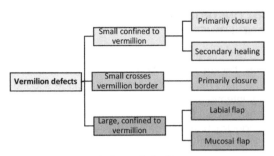

Fig. 5. Superficial defects of the lip.

primary closure is the simplest reconstruction technique.[5,32,41] Small lesions and scar of the vermilion can be excised in fusiform fashion and closed primarily.[42] Incisions should be placed in the radially oriented relaxing skin tension lines (RSTLs), and the mucocutaneous line should be avoided for optimal closure and cosmetic result.[2,27,42]

Primary closure may cause unpleasant redundant vermilion.[5] In a recent study, it was observed that mucosal advancement flaps resulted in better maintenance of the vermilion width compared with primary closure.[43]

Mucosal V-Y advancement
Small defect or volume deficiency of the vermilion may be restored using adjacent oral mucosa by V-Y advancement flaps movement (**Fig. 8**).[1,2]

Bocchi and colleagues[44] reports good results with no complications, such as vascular compromise, microstomia, retracted scars, or hypomobility, in restoration of vermilion in 16 patients by this technique. The advancement flap is created by a V-shaped incision to the level of the orbicularis oris with the apex of incision positioned toward the gingivolabial sulcus, creating an island flap

that is pedicled on the underlying deep tissue. The triangular-shaped island is advanced into the adjacent recipient site, maintaining sufficient deep-tissue attachments to ensure its viability. The donor site is closed primarily in a Y configuration. In some cases, horizontal movement is used using a single or bilateral opposing island flap.[1,2]

Mucosal advancement flap
The mucosal advancement flap is the most favored and common method for vermilion defect restoration.[1,25,34] It is indicated for repairing small defects isolated to the vermilion, diffuse actinic cheilitis, and subsequent reconstruction of a vermilionectomy of either lips.[3,24]

In this method, an incision is made along the vermilion border[3]; the labial mucosa is undermined in a plane deep to minor salivary glands and superficial to posterior surface of orbicularis oris muscle. The mucosal lining of the vestibule is mobilized and advanced forward to resurface the defect and remaining muscle (**Fig. 9**).[1–3]

Selective dissection techniques in an attempt to preserve the small neurovascular structure have been described. This technique is a one-stage surgery. Because the vermilion is modified mucosa, reconstruction with labial mucosa offers a very close substitute[1] with excellent aesthetic results.[1,45,46] Most patients regain some degree of sensation within months.[1]

The disadvantages of this technique are distortion of the anterior vermilion line caused by wound contraction, change in hair growth direction,[1] thinning of the lip, mucosal retraction,[3,24,32] decreased mucosal sensation,[47–49] color mismatch,[41,48] dryness, and excessive lip fullness from flap overadvancement.[4]

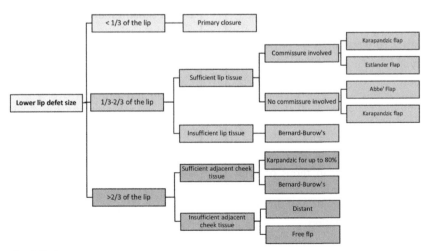

Fig. 6. Lower lip defects.

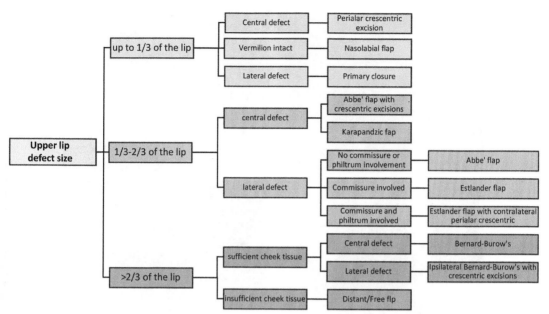

Fig. 7. Upper lip defects.

The limitations in this technique are the difficulty in reconstructing the fullness of the white roll because of scar contraction, difficulty in accurately repositioning the anterior vermilion line when there is a skin defect adjacent to lip margin,[1] and the inability to restore muscle bulk in defects involving the orbicularis-oris muscle.[5]

Mucosal cross lip flap
This flap is designed as a linear band of mucosa harvested from the vermilion or labial mucosa of the opposing lip and is used to restore the vermilion defect or add substance.[1,2,34] It is designed as a single pedicle flap or double pedicle (bucket handle) for reconstruction of a larger defect.[1]

The flap is usually dissected and elevated in the plane superficial to the muscle; however, the muscle and labial artery can be included. It is raised, rotated, and transferred across the oral aperture and sutured into the opposing vermilion defect. The donor site is closed primarily if it is the buccal vestibule or using a mucosal advancement at the vermilion (**Fig. 10**).[1,2,34] Division of the pedicle is performed after 2 to 3 weeks as the second stage.[1]

2-stage surgery, patient discomfort and restricted mouth opening are the disadvantages of this technique. Multiple other techniques are available using tongue flaps, vermilion advancement flaps, facial artery musculomucosal flaps, and cheek rotation flaps; but they are outside the

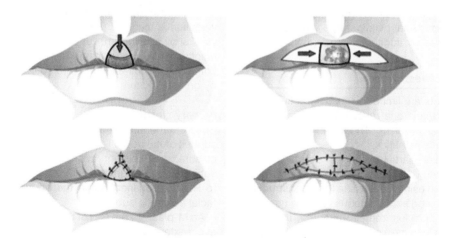

Fig. 8. Mucosal V-Y advancement. (*From* Weerda H. Reconstructive facial plastic surgery: a problem-solving manual. 1st edition. New York: Thieme; 2001; with permission.)

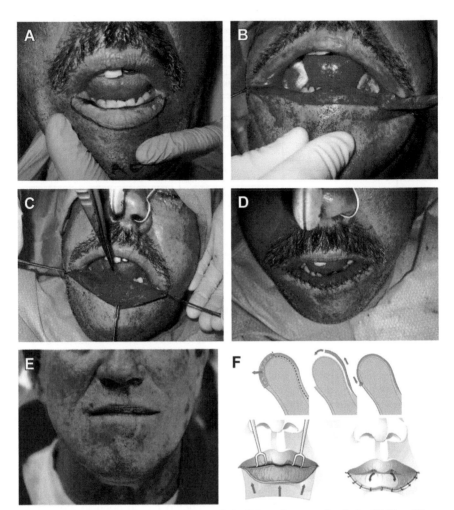

Fig. 9. (*A–F*) Mucosal advancement flap. (*A*) Outline of cheilitis and severe dysplasia. (*B*) Vermillion excision. (*C*) Labial mucosal advancement. (*D*) Closure. (*E*) Six months postoperatively. (*F*) Diagrammatical depiction. (*From [F] Weerda H. Reconstructive facial plastic surgery: a problem-solving manual. 1st edition. New York: Thieme; 2001; with permission.*)

scope of this article, and readers are recommended to review facial plastic surgery texts cited in the references for additional information.

Partial-Thickness Defect

These defects are limited to the tissue superficial to the orbicularis oris muscle and usually cause no functional problem. The basic challenge for the surgeon is esthetics.[34,41]

A perilabial partial-thickness defect can be closed primarily or with a variety of transposition flaps.[27] When using local tissue for reconstruction, only the skin and subcutaneous tissue is used and underlying muscles remain intact.[27] It is also preferred to confine tissue movement within the aesthetic region unless it causes distortion.[1] Conversion of partial-thickness defect to full thickness facilitates re-approximation, particularly when the vermilion is involved (**Fig. 11**).[35,50] A recent analysis shows excellent aesthetic and functional results when upper lip cutaneous defects were converted to full-thickness defects and repaired by primary closure.[51]

Primary closure

Small cutaneous defects in the lower lip and lateral subunit of the upper lip can be repaired by primary closure.[5,33] Excellent cosmetic results may be achieved by designing fusiform excisions parallel to RSTLs, confined within the boundaries of the facial aesthetic subunits.[1,34]

An M-plasty at the end of the excision is useful to avoid extension of the incision beyond the aesthetic borders. If the lesion crosses the vermilion, the incision must cross the mucocutaneous line at 90°.[31] In

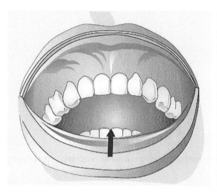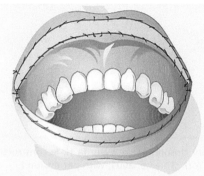

Fig. 10. Mucosal cross lip flap. The arrow shows the bipedicle flap being transferred to the upper lip. (*From* Weerda H. Reconstructive facial plastic surgery: a problem-solving manual. 1st edition. New York: Thieme; 2001; with permission.)

horizontal lesions, a Z-plasty may be used to disperse wounds and scars (**Fig. 12**).[2]

Cutaneous defects less than 50% of the width of philtrum may be reconstructed by primary closure; however, it can cause flattening of cupid's bow or an upward pull of the vermilion caused by wound contraction.[1]

Island advancement flap

Small to medium cutaneous defects involving lateral lips can be repaired by a subcutaneous island pedicled flap (**Fig. 13**).[33,52–56] These flaps are best to repair defects adjacent to the vermilion line.[34]

The flap is dissected down to the orbicularis oris muscle, maintaining a deep pedicle. The underlying facial musculature should not be violated. The flap is then advanced into the excision site and the donor site is closed in a V-Y fashion.[34] Some remaining normal skin may be removed in order to position the final scar into the nasal base or aesthetic boundaries.[33]

Intralabial transposition flap, labial rotational and advancement flap, melolabial transposition flap, and chin and submandibular transposition flap are also possible options but are outside the scope of this article; readers are recommended

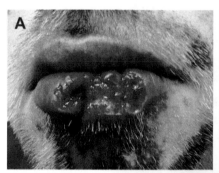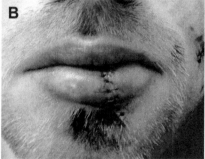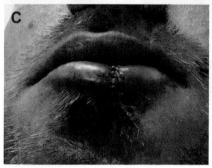

Fig. 11. (*A–C*) Primary closure of vermilion with conversion of partial thickness. (*A*) Partial-thickness dog bite. (*B, C*) Tissue undermined and closed primarily.

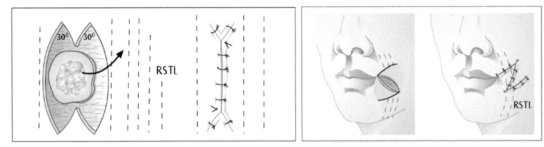

Fig. 12. Primary closure. (*From* Weerda H. Reconstructive facial plastic surgery: a problem-solving manual. 1st edition. New York: Thieme; 2001; with permission.)

to review facial plastic surgery texts cited in the references for additional information.

Full-Thickness Defect

Full-thickness defect reconstruction of the lips requires replacement of skin, muscle, mucosa, or a reasonable substitute and multilayer repair.[1] These defects have traditionally been classified according to the size and location of the defect.[34]

Small full-thickness defects: primary closure

Full-thickness defects that involve less than 30% (up to 50%[27,34]) of the stretched lower lip width or

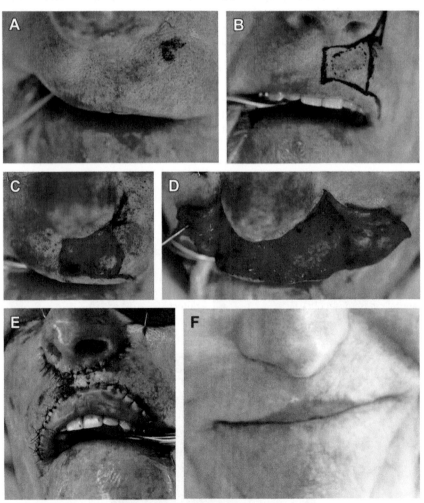

Fig. 13. Island advancement flap. (*A*) BCC upper lip. An 86-year-old man with multiple prior surgeries. (*B*) BCC demarcated with flaps outlined. (*C*) BCC excised. (*D*) Advancement flaps raised bilaterally. (*E*) Closure. (*F*) Six months postoperatively. Patient pleased with no desire for creation of cupid's bow.

25% of the upper lip width,[25] not including most of the philtral subunit, can be removed by wedge excision or its variants and repaired by primary layered closure[3,24,57] without causing significant microstomia.[32] The size rules are especially applicable to elderly patients with greater tissue laxity.[34]

A recent study by Soliman and colleagues[58] shows superior functional and aesthetic results obtained with primary closure. The investigators suggested that local flaps are often overused. They advocate primary closure of defects that comprise 40% of the upper lip and 50% of the lower lip.

Optimal primary repair of full-thickness defects requires the approximation of at least 4 tissue layers: mucosa, muscle, subcutaneous tissue, and skin epithelium.[1] The anterior vermilion line is the principal landmark of the lip, and its location at the edge of the wound needs to be identified and marked before incision to avoid distortion during injection and dissection. Meticulous closure of the vermilion is critical, both anteriorly and posteriorly, to prevent asymmetry.[27] Early approximation of the vermilion border is recommended as a guide for closure of the other layers and maximizes the cosmetic outcome.[1,27] Precise anastomosis of the orbicularis oris muscle ends is important to reconstitute the oral sphincter and prevent notched or retracted vermilion.[1,32] Aesthetic wound closure can be achieved by undermining the skin and mucosal edge of the wound and closure of epithelium with slight skin eversion.[1,32,33,59] A Z-plasty may be combined with design or performed as a secondary procedure.

A *V-shape (wedge) excision* (**Fig. 14**) is the most common and simplest method to repair small lip defects and malignancies.[1,3] The wedge resection is designed with the incisions perpendicular to the red lip, tapered as they enter the white lip.[5] The excision is parallel to RSTLs, which are oriented vertically in the central portion and skewed in the lateral region of lip.[1,27]

Calhoun[60] has reported that classic V excision can cause a noticeable step-off in the vermilion-cutaneous junction. He showed that a slight angulation of the lateral incision allows for precise matching of the vermilion-cutaneous junction.[6]

The apex of the wedge should not exceed 30° and not cross the mental crease to avoid a conspicuous cutaneous deformity and scar. If both of these conditions cannot be met, another modification, such as a W- or U-shape design, should be used.[3,27] A vermilionectomy can be performed at the same time as the wedge excision (**Fig. 15**). Attention should be given to the alignment of the vermilion and orbicularis muscle.

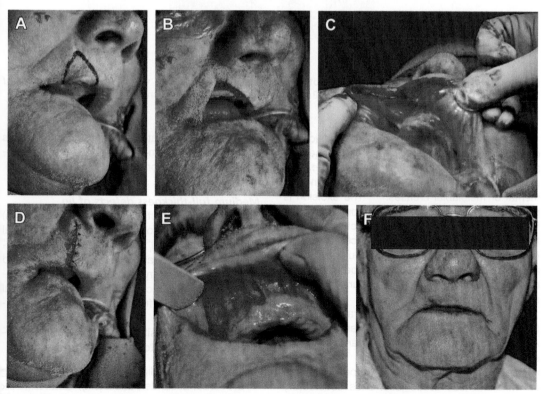

Fig. 14. (*A–F*) Wedge excision upper lip with primary closure. (*E, F*) Patient 3 months postoperatively.

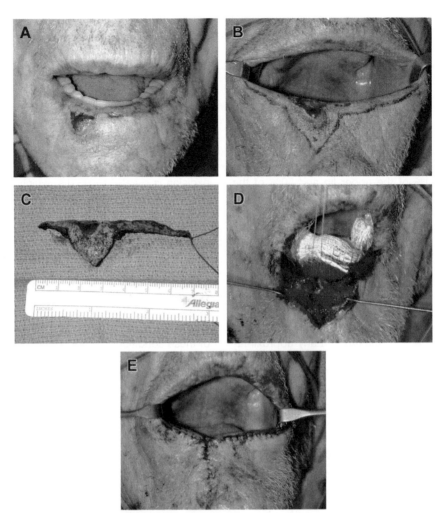

Fig. 15. (*A–E*) Primary closure. Combination of V-shape (wedge) excision and vermilionectomy. (*Courtesy of* David E. Urbanek, DMD, MS, and Jonathan S. Bailey, DMD, MD, FACS, Carle Foundation Hospital, Urbana, IL.)

A *W-shaped* (**Fig. 16**) excision is a modification of a wedge excision that allows greater resection and preserves the integrity of the aesthetic subunit[24] without extending the incisions beyond the mental or melolabial creases.[1,27] The excision is planned, with the apices of the W oriented away from the vermilion border with each angle less than 30°.[3] In laterally located defects, the angle formed by the lateral subunit should be larger and more obliquely oriented to properly align the closure and achieve a more natural-appearing scar.[1,24,27,47]

W-plasty can be used for moderate-sized defects up to one-third of the lower lip width.[3] Aesthetic results in the upper lip are often less satisfactory, in part, because of the specific aesthetic subunits and that the upper lip is able to withstand less tissue loss. Less satisfactory aesthetic result is particularly noticeable in mid-

upper lip defects at the philtrum and cupid's bow.[33] Again, a vermilionectomy can be incorporated into the excision.

Medium full-thickness defects of lip

Medium-sized defects (30%–60% of lip length) represent the most complex challenges in surgical planning.[27] Although primary closure of this defects of this size is feasible, it is not recommended because of secondary wound tension and microstomia.[41] These defects require some form of local flap to borrow tissue from the opposing lip or adjacent tissue.[4,6]

Depending on the site of the defect, 2 major techniques are available to reconstruct these defects:

I. Lip switch/cross lip flap (3 most common are the Abbe, Estlander, and Stein)
II. Circumoral advancement or rotational flap

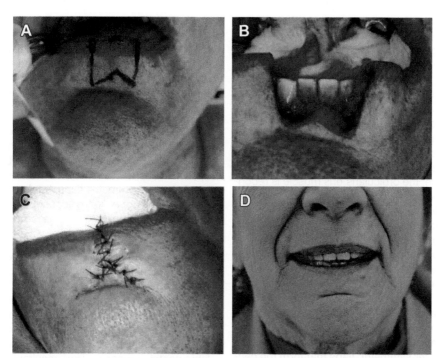

Fig. 16. (*A*) SCC lower lip. (*B*) W-wedge excision. (*C*) Closure. (*D*) Six months postoperatively.

(I.A) Abbe flap Cross-lip transfer of full-thickness tissue was described first by Sabattini (1838) and later by Abbe in 1898.[11,12,61,62] It is designed as a rotational or lip switch flap from the opposite lip, based on the labial artery, which is preserved on one side to serve as a pedicle of the interpolated flap. There is no associated vein, and venous drainage is provided by small veins that parallel the course of the artery.[1,3,27,47]

Although this flap was initially designed to correct midline defects of the upper lip,[48] it has been used for reconstruction of full-thickness defects affecting 30% to 60%[5] of the width of either lip medial to the commissure (**Fig. 17**).[1,2,5]

The donor site is traditionally designed similar to the V-shaped full-thickness excision; but it can also be designed to accommodate different variations, such as W shape or rectangle, depending on the defect situation. This flap is designed conventionally as the same height and half of the width of the defect[1,62] to achieve a proportional reduction in size of both lips.[27] However, the size of the flaps may range from one that is the size of a given defect to one that fills only a small portion of the defect.[1] The flap is created by a full-thickness incision with preservation of the labial artery on the medial or lateral pedicle within the vermilion. Approximately 5 mm of vermilion mucosa should be preserved for adequate blood supply.[5] The pedicle should be place at the defect midpoint. The flap is rotated 180° as it is inserted into the opposing lip defect and closed in multiple layers.

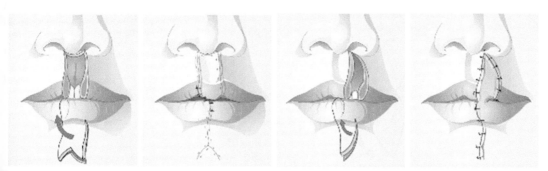

Fig. 17. Abbe flap. (*From* Weerda H. Reconstructive facial plastic surgery: a problem-solving manual. 1st edition. New York: Thieme; 2001; with permission.)

The donor site is repaired primarily. Patients are placed on a liquid or soft diet for the period of vascular ingrowth. In approximately 3 weeks, the pedicle on the vermilion is divided and the flap inset.[1,4,34]

A cross-lip flap can be combined with unilateral or bilateral advancement flaps to reconstruct major tissue loss.[1] Bilateral Abbe flaps are advised for large central defects of the lower lip to avoid upper lip asymmetry.[5]

In this technique, the defect is repaired with similar tissue; the orbicularis oris muscle is reconstructed; the continuity of the circumoral sphincter is reestablished[24]; and the commissure is not violated. Adequate sensory and voluntary motor function is regained.[63–67]

The major disadvantages are damage to the artery on elevation of the flap, relative microstomia, 2-stage surgery, risk of injuring the flap by opening the mouth, prolonged phase of denervation, and thickened appearance caused by scar and trapdoor deformity.

The Stein flap is essentially a double Abbe flap. It has 2 smaller symmetric flaps that form the central portion of the upper lip to reconstruct the lower lip. This flap is a complicated and less-favored flap.

(I.B) Estlander This design was described by Estlander in 1872.[67] It is a cross-lip flap. It is similar to the Abbe flap but has its point of rotation at the commissure (**Fig. 18**). It is designed for repairing a defect involving the oral commissure of either lips and transfers a full-thickness lip flap around the oral commissure on a small medially vascular pedicle containing the labial artery.[1,27,61,67] In contrast to the Abbe flap, it is a single-stage reconstruction.[4,33,67]

The flap design is similar to the Abbe flap; its dimension is equivalent in height and half the width of the defect. It is usually designed as a triangle but can be modified to lie within the melolabial crease to reduce scarring.[1,4]

The major disadvantages of this flap are a blunted oral commissure[1] and prolonged denervation (lasting 6–18 months).[3] The blunted commissure frequently diminishes over time,[25] and revision commissuroplasty is rarely required.[4,24,68]

(I.C) In 1848, Stein described a method of reconstructing the lower lip with 2 flaps from the center of the upper lip hinged on the labial vessels.[69] The Stein flap is essentially a double Abbe flap. It has 2 smaller symmetric flaps that form the central portion of the upper lip to reconstruct the lower lip. This flap is a complicated and less-favored flap.

(II.A) Bilateral lip advancement Full-thickness defects, measuring up to one-half of the lower lip,[6,33] may be reconstructed with unilateral or bilateral lip advancement (**Fig. 19**).[1,3,6,27]

In this technique, the wide, rectangular wedge of the tissue is excised. Unilateral or bilateral full-thickness advancement flaps are created by an inferior arc shape releasing the incision along the labiomental crease.[3] The resultant flaps are advanced medially around the mental prominence to close the defect. Incisional release at the commissure or removal of crescents around the mental prominence incision may be necessary to mobilize the flap.[3]

In the upper lip, soft tissue attachment to the underlying bony skeleton limits compensatory movement of the remaining lip. A perialar excision as described by Webster[70] minimizes this effect by allowing the lateral lip elements to be advanced.

Central upper lip defects up to two-thirds of the lip width may be reconstructed with perialar crescentic advancement flaps combined with an Abbe flap to restore the philtral subunit.[6,20] Although this technique causes lip tightness, this improves over time and provides a satisfactory cosmetic result.[27]

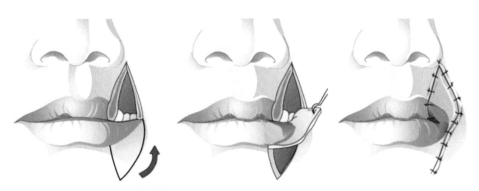

Fig. 18. Estlander. (*From* Weerda H. Reconstructive facial plastic surgery: a problem-solving manual. 1st edition. New York: Thieme; 2001; with permission.)

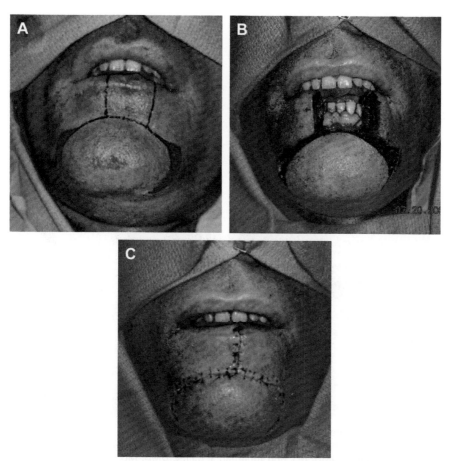

Fig. 19. Bilateral lip advancement (lower lip)/Fernandes flap. (*A*) Flap design. (*B*) Full-thickness defect, with excision of skin and subcutaneous tissue for advancement of flaps. (*C*) Closed in layers; scar in labiomental crease. (*Courtesy of* Phillip Pirgousis, MBBS, BDS, FRCS, FRACDS, University of Florida College of Medicine-Jacksonville, Jacksonville, FL, and Rui Fernandes MD, DMD, FACS, University of Florida College of Medicine-Jacksonville, Jacksonville, FL.)

(II.B) Stair step design Johanson and colleagues[71] proposed the stair-step design flap in 1974 for a defect that is too wide to close directly but not wide enough to require transfer tissue by other flap designs (**Fig. 20**). This design is ideally suited for smaller defects but is capable of reconstructing a defect involving one-half to two-thirds of the lower lip.[24,33]

In this method, the lower lip lesion is resected using a rectangular-shaped excision. A series of 2 to 4 of connected bilateral small rectangular are excised (skin and subcutaneous tissue only) in a downward diagonal fashion at a 45° angle, following the aesthetic border of the chin.[24,72] At the termination of the incisions, bilateral, small triangles are excised. This design allows the advancement of the flap in the direction of the defect. As the lip segments are advanced, the series of rectangular and terminal triangles are closed, creating a stair-step wound closure line. This advancement flap can be used unilaterally for lateral defects or bilaterally to close central defects.[73]

Several advantages of this technique are minimized scar contracture,[1] unchanged muscle fibers direction, preserved innervation and vascularity of the flap owing to its broad pedicle, and intact commissures.[3]

The main drawback is a geometric scar that is unnatural to the lower face and does not follow the mental crease.[1,33]

(II.C) Gillies fan flap This flap is a rotation-advancement flap that was initially described by Gillies and Millard in 1957.[17]

It is a modification of the technique described by von Bruns[74] and is designed to transfer the remaining lip segment from one side of a defect together with the lateral portion of the opposing lip[1,27] around the commissure in the same fashion as Estlander.[24,25,75] It is based on the

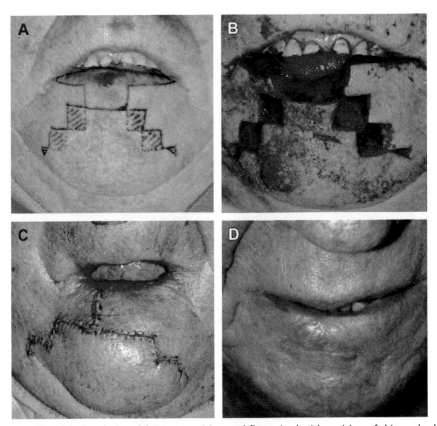

Fig. 20. Stair step flap. (*A*) Flap design. (*B*) Tumor excision and flap raised with excision of skin and subcutaneous tissue at each step. (*C*) Closure in layers. (*D*) Three weeks postoperatively. Scar will flatten and fade with time. (*Courtesy of* David E. Urbanek, DMD, MS, and Jonathan S. Bailey, DMD, MD, FACS, Carle Foundation Hospital, Urbana, IL.)

superior labial artery[27] and has a narrow pedicle.[1]

This composite flap is created by full-thickness lip incisions from the inferior aspect of the defect, which extends laterally around the commissure and superiorly into the melolabial fold,[4,40] essentially paralleling the orbicularis-oris. A secondary incision is made toward the superior vermilion without compromising the superior labial artery. Then the flap is rotated and advanced to close the defect, and the layer closure is performed (**Fig. 21**).

The advantages of this technique are more available tissue from the nasolabial region, one-stage reconstruction surgery, and maintained orbicularis-oris continuity. The primary limitations

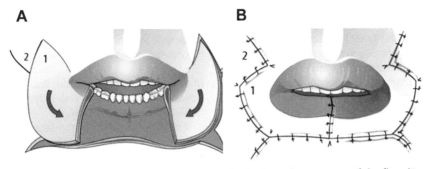

Fig. 21. Gillies fan flap. 1 and 2, Z-plasty is incorporated to the facilitated movement of the flap. (*From* Weerda H. Reconstructive facial plastic surgery: a problem-solving manual. 1st edition. New York: Thieme; 2001; with permission.)

of this approach are microstomia, blunted commissure, and vermilion deficiency.[25] Because the orbicularis is not fully dissected, full function and sensation may not return and oral incompetence may also result[3,4,24]; however, partial reinnervation seems to occur in 12 to 18 months.[24,47,76,77]

The Gillies flap can be used bilaterally or in combination with other flaps to restore large full-thickness lip defects of up to 80% of the lip. Z-plasty may be incorporated to the facilitated movement of the flap.[2]

(II.D) McGregor flap McGregor has modified the Gillies technique to reconstruct upper lip defects.[1] It is a rectangular composite flap, based on the labial artery, created by a full-thickness lip incision and transfers the tissue from the melolabial region to the defect of the upper lip.

It is indicated for reconstruction of lateral upper lip defect when there is not sufficient tissue without recruitment of cheek tissue. This technique fails to reconstruct the muscle of the sphincter and the vermilion. It needs to be combined by other techniques such as mucosal advancement to reconstruct the vermilion. It can be used bilaterally for large upper lip full-thickness defects.[1]

(II.E) Karapandzic flap The circumoral advancement-rotation flap initially described by von Bruns in 1857 (**Fig. 22**).[24] He used a full-thickness flap to rotate the upper lip and perioral tissue down and around to reconstruct the lower lip defect, which resulted in denervation of the orbicularis oris muscle.[24,74]

In 1974, Karapandzic[19,24,78] modified von Bruns' technique. In his modification, the incisional design was identical to the original technique; but a full-thickness flap was not created, and the neurovascular supply of the lip was preserved via meticulous dissection,[6,24] so optimal oral competence, sensory, and function were preserved.

The flap is created by circumoral incisions extended bilaterally from the base of the defect to the upper lips by placing incisions in the mental and nasolabial crease.[24] The thickness of the flaps should be maintained relatively constant throughout their length. Neurovascular bundles are identified, bluntly dissected, and preserved. The dissection of peripheral muscle fibers allows advancement without dissection of the mucosa.[25] The mucosa is incised only if needed.[4] The flap is advanced, and the layer closure is performed.

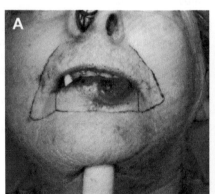
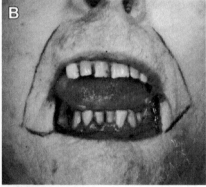
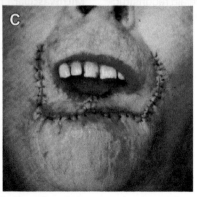

Fig. 22. Karapandzic flap. (*A*) Flap design. Along labiomental crease. (*B*) Resulting lip defect. (*C*) Flaps medially advanced and closed in layers. (*Courtesy of* David E. Urbanek, DMD, MS, and Jonathan S. Bailey, DMD, MD, FACS, Carle Foundation Hospital, Urbana, IL.)

This method is usually used to reconstruct defects involving up to two-thirds of the lower lip and, to a lesser degree, the upper lip. Some investigators state it can be designed bilaterally to reconstruct defects of up to 80% of the total lip length.[24,25,47,76,79,80] It is useful in cases whereby radiation had been previously used and blood supply is compromised.[6]

The technique has predictable results, with superior function, sensation, and cosmetic outcome.[4,24] It causes blunting of the commissure and some degree of microstomia[4,24]; however, secondary correction of the mouth opening is seldom needed.[33]

Large full-thickness defect

Total lip reconstruction presents the biggest functional and cosmetic reconstruction challenge for surgeons.[4,27] The defects usually involve the lower lip. Defects greater than two-thirds of the lip need transfer of adjacent cheek tissue or tissue from distant sites to prevent microstomia.[1] If there is a lack of residual lip tissue, microvascular free tissue transfer must be considered.[4] Potential complications of total lip reconstruction include hypertrophic scarring, disfigurement, loss of sensation, microstomia, loss of oral competence, and loss of natural gingivobuccal sulcus. These complications can make denture placement challenging.

Bilateral cheek advancement flaps (Bernard–von Burow) Bernard (1852)[16] and von Burow[15] (1853) separately described bilateral horizontal cheek advancement.

This advancement is performed by a horizontal full- or partial-thickness incision[4] extended laterally from the commissure and excision of the skin and subcutaneous triangles (von Burow triangles[33]) at the superior and inferior margin of the flap to facilitate advancement.

Upper lip reconstruction is accomplished with the excision of 4 triangles and lower lip reconstruction with the excision of 3 triangles (**Fig. 23**).[27] The remaining orbicularis muscle is freed up to allow for flap advancement.[1]

This technique was originally described as full-thickness excisions but was later modified and performed as cutaneous and mucosal excisions and flap dissection to minimize disruption of the facial structure[28,33] and preserve sensory innervation.

It is technically difficult, and oral function is fair at best.[1] It fails to restore the vermilion and needs to be combined with other techniques, such as a buccal mucosal flap or tongue flap, to reconstruct the missing vermilion.[4] This technique is better suited for upper lip reconstruction because of less risk for the development of postoperative oral incompetence.

Webster technique In 1960, Webster and colleagues[81] described the modification of Bernard–von Burow for the reconstruction of the lower lip by using a more linear horizontal advancement of the cheek, placing scar lines in natural facial skin creases and avoiding the violation of the aesthetic region of the chin (**Fig. 24**).[1] Webster and colleagues recommended placement of triangular excisions along the nasolabial fold with excision only through skin and subcutaneous tissue. This design minimizes the tendency for vertical deficiency of the lower lip[1,81] and provides better muscle function.

Distant flap Distant flaps are used if adjacent local tissue is unavailable owing to trauma or extensive disease involvement.[3,82] Flaps from the scalp and forehead and submandibular, deltopectoral, pectoralis-major, sternocleidomastoid, and cervicodeltopectoral flaps have been described in literature.[27,33,47,83] These flaps provide tissue for wound closure and lip restoration; but compared with local techniques, they are not capable of restoring adequate function and satisfactory cosmetics.[27,33]

Microvascular reconstruction Microvascular reconstruction allows for single-stage reconstruction of large defects[27] with high success rates and good functional and cosmetic results (**Fig. 25**).[84,85]

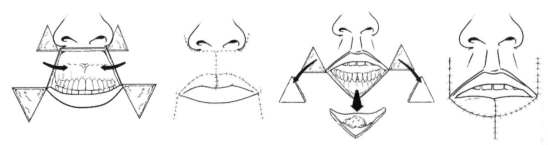

Fig. 23. Bilateral cheek advancement flaps (Bernard–von Burow). (*From* Coppit GL, Lin DT, Burkey BB. Current concepts in lip reconstruction. Curr Opin Otolaryngol Head Neck Surg 2004;12:281–7; with permission.)

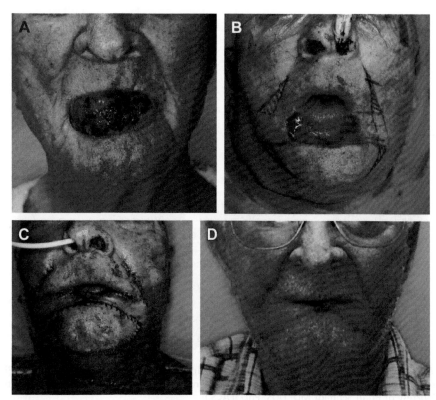

Fig. 24. (*A–D*) Webster Technique. (*A*) Large SCC. (*B*) Resection with flap design. The crescents are areas of skin and subcutaneous tissue that will be excised for flap advancement. (*C*) Closure: note the microstomia that will improve with time. (*D*) Postoperative results a few weeks later. (*Courtesy of* David E. Urbanek, DMD, MS, and Jonathan S. Bailey, DMD, MD, FACS, Carle Foundation Hospital, Urbana, IL.)

The most commonly used free flap to reconstruct total or near-total lip defect is the radial forearm free flap. It may also be transferred along with the palmaris longus tendon, which anchors to the orbicularis muscle and/or modiolus to function as a sling between 2 commissures and to provide static support for oral competence.[4,28,33,86] It may also be fashioned to the nasolabial or malar periosteum. Alternatively, the flexor carpi radialis tendon or a nonvascularized folded fascia lata graft can be used as a sling over which the radial forearm flap is draped.[33] This flap may be transferred as a sensate free flap by performing anastomosis of the lateral antebrachial cutaneous nerve to the mental nerve to restore some competence and sensation, which was first described by Sakai and colleagues in 1989.[87]

Free flaps not only provide reconstruction of soft tissue but can also provide bone if there is bone involvement with an osteofasciocutaneous flap.[27] Fibula flap or iliac crest flap based on deep circumflex iliac vessels offer the best reconstruction method for the anterior mandible defect.[33]

Other microvascular approaches including the gracilis free flap[88] for total lower lip reconstruction

and temporal scalp free flap for upper lip defects have also been described.[89]

Commissuroplasty Finally, the Estlander cross-lip flap and other methods can cause blunting and distortion of lip commissures and shortening of the oral fissure that require secondary correction.[1,2]

The simplest method of commissureplasty (Converse 1959, Weerda 1983)[2,90] involves making a horizontal full-thickness incision at the level of the blunted commissure, in the direction of the oral fissure, which extends laterally to the point corresponding in position of the contralateral normal commissure. The epithelium above and below the incision is removed; the labial mucosa is then mobilized and advanced forward on each side of the incision to restore a vermilion surface.[47,91]

Gillies and Millard[17] (1957) described excising a triangular segment of skin lateral to the rounded commissure, raising and rotating a vermilion flap from the lower (or upper) lip to reconstruct the opposite vermilion and mobilizing a mucosal flap to form the vermilion of the other lip.[2]

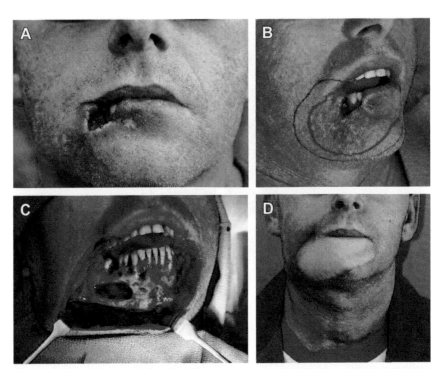

Fig. 25. (A–D) Radial forearm free flap. (A) Large SCC lower lip. Note induration and ulceration. (B) Planned excision. (C) Resection including entire periosteum and right mental nerve. (D) Final reconstruction 3 weeks postoperatively. (Courtesy of Brian Schmidt MD, DDS, PhD, FACS.)

SUMMARY

Lips are complex and highly functional components that are located in an esthetic area of the face. The complexity of the lip structure leads to a complex functional unit that is critical in maintaining one's quality of life.

The unique anatomy and the location of the lips bring specific challenges to the reconstructive surgeon. Cancer lesions, trauma, or burns cause most common defects of the lips. Repairing these defects requires a clear understanding of anatomy, pathology, patients' factors, and surgical techniques.

Size, location, and thickness of the lesion are the most important determining factors to choose the proper surgical approach. Smaller defects can be repaired by primary reconstruction, followed by a local flap from the remaining labial or adjacent tissue. Larger defects may need a distant tissue flap or free flap. The ultimate goal in lip reconstruction is to reach a high level of esthetics while attempting to maintain normal function.

REFERENCES

1. Renner GJ. Reconstruction of the lip 475-524. In: Baker SR, editor. Local flaps in facial reconstruction. 2nd edition. Philadelphia: Mosby; 2007.

2. Weerda H. Reconstructive facial plastic surgery: a problem-solving manual. 1st edition. Thieme; 2001.

3. McCarn KE, Park SS. Lip reconstruction. Otolaryngol Clin North Am 2007;40:361–80.

4. Anvar BA, Evans BC, Evans GR. Lip reconstruction. Plast Reconstr Surg 2007;120(4):57e–64e.

5. Ishii LE, Byrne PJ. Lip reconstruction. Facial Plast Surg Clin North Am 2009;17(3):445–53.

6. Cupp CL, Larrabee WF. Reconstruction of the lip. Oper Tech Otolaryngol–Head Neck Surg 1993; 4(1):46–53.

7. Williams EF, Hove C. Lip reconstruction. Chapter 51. In: Paper ID, Holt GR, Larrabee WF, et al, editors. Facial plastic and reconstructive surgery. 2nd edition. New York: Thieme; 2002.

8. Hauben DJ. Sushruta Samhita (Sushruta's collection) (800-600 B.C ?) Pioneer of plastic surgery. Acta Chir Plast 1984;26:65–8.

9. Dieffenbach JF. Die operative chirurgie, vol. 1. Leipzig (Germany): Brockhaus; 1845. p. 423. Medscape.

10. Dieffenbach JF. Chirurgische Erfahrungen, bensonders uber die Wiederherstellung Zerstoerter Theile des Menschlichen Koerpers nach Neuen Methoden. Berlin: TCF Enslin; 1829. p. 34. Medscape.

11. Sabattini P. Cenno storico dell-origine e progresso della rinoplastica e cheiloplastica seguito dalla

descrizione di queste operazioni sopra un solo individuo. Bologna: Balla Arti; 1838. Medscape.

12. Abbe R. A new plastic operation for the relief of deformity due to double harelip. Med Rec 1898; 53:447. Medscape.

13. Estlander JA. Methode d'autoplastie de la joue ou d'une levre par un lambeau emprunte a l'autre levre. Rev Mens Med Chir 1877;1:344. Medscape.

14. Estlander JA. Eine Methode, aus der einen Lippe Substanzverluste der anderen zu ersetzen. Archiv fur klinische Chirurgie 1872;14:622.

15. Bernard C. Cancer de la levre inferieure opere par un procede nouveau. Bull Mem Soc Chir Paris 1853;3:357.

16. Mazzola RF, Lupo G. Evolving concepts in lip reconstruction. Clin Plast Surg 1984;11(4): 583–617.

17. Gillies HD, Millard DR Jr. Principles and art of plastic surgery. Boston: Little Brown; 1957.

18. Sajjadian A, Narayan D. Lip reconstruction procedure. Medscape. Available at: http://emedicine. medscape.com/article/1288447-overview#a0101.

19. Karapandzic M. Reconstruction of lip defects by local arterial flaps. Br J Plast Surg 1974;27(1): 93–7.

20. Carty MJ, Pribaz JJ. Lip and cheek reconstruction. In: Siemionow MZ, Eisenmann-Klein M, editors. Plastic and reconstructive surgery, London: Springer specialist surgery series. 2010.

21. Harii K, Ohmori K, Torii S. Free gracilis muscle transplantation, with microneurovascular anastomoses for the treatment of facial paralysis. A preliminary report. Plast Reconstr Surg 1976;57(2):133–43.

22. Devauchelle B, Badet L, Lengele B, et al. First human face allograft: early report. Lancet 2006;368: 203–9.

23. Dubernard JM, Lengele B, Morelon E, et al. Outcomes 18 months after the first human partial face transplantation. N Engl J Med 2007;357(24): 2451–60.

24. Neligan PC. Cheek and lip reconstruction. In: Neligan PC, editor. Plastic surgery. vol. 6. 3rd edition.

25. Neligan PC. Strategies in lip reconstruction. Clin Plast Surg 2009;36:477–85.

26. Jahan-Parwar B, Meyers AD, et al. Lips and Perioral Region Anatomy, Medscape. Available at: http:// emedicine.medscape.com/article/835209-overview #aw2aab6b5.

27. Coppit GL, Lin DT, Burkey BB. Current concepts in lip reconstruction. Curr Opin Otolaryngol Head Neck Surg 2004;12:281–7.

28. Shah JP, Patel SG, Singh B. Lips Chapter 7. In: Shah JP, Patel SG, Singh B, editors. Jatin shah's head and neck surgery and oncology. 4th edition. Philadelphia: Mosby; 2012.

29. Abreu L, Kruger E, Tennant M. Lip cancer in Western Australia, 1982-2006: a 25-year retrospective epidemiological study. Aust Dent J 2009;54:130–5.

30. Molnar L, Ronay P, Tapolcsanyi L. Carcinoma of the lip. Analysis of the material of 25 years. Oncology 1974;29:101–21.

31. Wilson JS, Walker EP. Reconstruction of the lower lip. Head Neck Surg 1981;4:29–44.

32. Lubek JE, Ord RA. Lip reconstruction. Oral Maxillofacial Surg Clin North Am 2013;25:203–14.

33. Vuyk HD, Leemans CR. Lip reconstruction. In: Vuyk HD, Lohuis PJ, editors. Facial plastic and reconstructive surgery. 1st edition. London: Hodder Arnold; 2006.

34. Harris L, Higgins K, Enepekides D. Local flap reconstruction of acquired lip defects. Curr Opin Otolaryngol Head Neck Surg 2012;20:254–61.

35. Pepper JP, Baker SR. Local flaps: cheek and lip reconstruction. JAMA Facial Plast Surg 2013; 15(5):374–82.

36. Gloster HM Jr. The use of second-intention healing for partial-thickness Mohs defects involving the vermilion and/or mucosal surfaces of the lip. J Am Acad Dermatol 2002;47(6):893–7.

37. Becker GD, Adams LA, Levin BC. Outcome analysis of Mohs surgery of the lip and chin: comparing secondary intention healing and surgery. Laryngoscope 1995;105(11):1176–83.

38. Zitelli JA. Wound healing by secondary intention. A cosmetic appraisal. J Am Acad Dermatol 1983; 9(3):407–15.

39. Leonard AL, Hanke CW. Second intention healing for intermediate and large postsurgical defects of the lip. J Am Acad Dermatol 2007; 57(5):832–5.

40. McCarn KE, Park SS. Lip reconstruction. Facial Plast Surg Clin North Am 2005;13(2):301–14.

41. Malard O, Corre P, Jégoux F, et al. Surgical repair of labial defect. Eur Ann Otorhinolaryngol Head Neck Dis 2010;127(2):49–62.

42. Galyon SW, Frodel JL. Lip and perioral defects. Otolaryngol Clin North Am 2001;34:647–66.

43. Sand M, Altmeyer P, Bechara FG. Mucosal advancement flap versus primary closure after vermilionectomy of the lower lip. Dermatol Surg 2010; 36:1987–92.

44. Bocchi A, Baccarani A, Bianco G, et al. Double V-Y advancement flap in the management of lower lip reconstruction. Ann Plast Surg 2003; 51:205.

45. Manstein CH. Vermilionectomy and mucosal advancement. Plast Reconstr Surg 1997;100(5):1363.

46. Ay A, Aytekin A. Meshing technique in mucosal advancement flaps for vermilionectomy defects. Plast Reconstr Surg 2003;112:1739–40.

47. Renner G. Reconstruction of the lip. In: Baker SR, Swanson N, editors. Local flaps in facial reconstruction. New York: Mosby; 1995. p. 345–96.

48. Krunic AL, Weitzul S, Taylor RS, et al. Advanced reconstructive techniques for the lip and perioral area. Dermatol Clin 2005;23:43–53, v–vi.

49. Neligan P, Gullane P, Werning J. Lip reconstruction. In: Werning J, editor. Oral cancer. New York: Thieme Medical Publishing Inc; 2006. p. 180–93.

50. Baker SR. In: Baker SR, editor. Flap classification and design: local flaps in facial reconstruction. 2nd edition. St Louis (MO): CV Mosby; 2007. p. 71–106.

51. Godek CP, Weinzweig J, Bartlett SP. Lip reconstruction following Mohs' surgery: the role for composite resection and primary closure. Plast Reconstr Surg 2000;106(4):798–804.

52. Skouge JW. Upper lip repair - the subcutaneous pedicle flap. J Dermatol Surg Oncol 1990;16:63–8.

53. Griffin GR, Weber S, Baker SR. Outcomes following V-Y advancement flap reconstruction of large upper lip defects. Arch Facial Plast Surg 2012;14(3):193–7.

54. Rustad TJ, Hartshorn DO, Clevens RA, et al. The subcutaneous pedicle flap in melolabial reconstruction. Arch Otolaryngol Head Neck Surg 1998;124(10):1163–6.

55. Zook EG, Van Beek AL, Russell RC, et al. V-Y advancement flap for facial defects. Plast Reconstr Surg 1980;65(6):786–97.

56. Herbert DC, Harrison RG. Nasolabial subcutaneous pedicle flaps. Br J Plast Surg 1975;28(2):85–9.

57. Langstein H, Robb G. Lip and perioral reconstruction. Clin Plast Surg 2005;32:431–45.

58. Soliman S, Hatef DA, Hollier LH Jr, et al. The rationale for direct linear closure of facial Mohs' defects. Plast Reconstr Surg 2011;127:142–9.

59. McGregor IA. Lips. In: McGregor IA, Howard DJ, editors. Rob & Smith's operative surgery. 4th edition. Part I: head and neck. Oxford (United Kingdom): Butterworth-Heinemann; 1992. p. 105–23.

60. Calhoun K. Reconstruction of small and medium sized defects of the lower lip. Am J Otol 1992;13:16–22.

61. Mazzola RF, Hueston JT. A forgotten innovator in facial reconstruction: Pietro Sabattini. Plast Reconstr Surg 1990;85(4):621–6.

62. Agostini T. The Sabattini-Abbé flap: a historical note. Plast Reconstr Surg 2009;123(2):767.

63. Smith JW. Anatomical and physiologic acclimatization of tissue transplanted by the lip switch technique. Plast Reconstr Surg 1960;26:40.

64. Thompson N, Pollard AC. Motor function in Abbe flaps: a histochemical study of motor reinnervation in transplanted muscle tissue of the lip in man. Br J Plast Surg 1961;14:66.

65. Burget G, Menick F. Aesthetic restoration of one-half of the upper lip. Plast Reconstr Surg 1986;78:583–93.

66. Abbe R. A new plastic operation for the relief of deformity due to double harelip. Plast Reconstr Surg 1968;42:481–3.

67. Estlander J. Eine methode aus er einen ippe substanzverluste der anderen zu ersetzein. Arch Klin Chir 1872;14:622 [Reprinted in English in Plast Reconstr Surg 1968;42:361–6].

68. Kroll S. Lip reconstruction. In: Kroll SS, editor. Reconstructive plastic surgery for cancer. St Louis (MO): Mosby Year Book; 1996. p. 201–9.

69. Stein SA. Lip repair (cheiloplasty) performed by a new method. Hosp-Meddel 1848;1:212. [Reprinted in Plast Reconstr Surg 53:332, 1974.]

70. Webster J. Crescentic peri-alar cheek excision for upper lip flap advancement with a short history of upper lip repair. Plast Reconstr Surg 1955;16:434–64.

71. Johanson B, Aspelund E, Breine U, et al. Surgical treatment of non-traumatic lower lip lesions with special reference to the step technique: a follow up on 149 patients. Scand J Plast Reconstr Surg 1974;8:232–40.

72. Sullivan D. "Staircase" closure of lower lip defects. Ann Plast Surg 1978;1:392–7.

73. Zide BM. Deformities of the lip and cheeks. In: McCarthy JG, editor. Plastic surgery, vol. 3. Philadelphia: W.B.Saunders; 1990. p. 2009–56.

74. Hauben DJ. Victor von Bruns (1812-1883) and his contributions to plastic and reconstructive surgery. Plast Reconstr Surg 1985;75(1):120–7.

75. McGregor IA. Reconstruction of the lower lip. Br J Plast Surg 1983;36(1):40–7.

76. Ducic Y, Athre R, Cochran CS, et al. The split orbicularis myomucosal flap for lower lip reconstruction. Arch Facial Plast Surg 2005;7:347–52.

77. Rea JL, Davis WE, Rittenhouse LK, et al. Reinnervation of an Abbe-Estlander and a Gillies fan flap of the lower lip: electromyographic comparison. Arch Otolaryngol 1978;104:294–5.

78. Ethunandan M, Macpherson DW, Santhanam V. Karapandzic flap for reconstruction of lip defects. J Oral Maxillofac Surg 2007;65(12):2512–7.

79. Williams E, Hove C. Lip reconstruction. In: Papel I, editor. Facial plastic and reconstructive surgery. New York: Thieme; 2002. p. 634–45.

80. Eguchi T, Nakatsuka T, Mori Y, et al. Total reconstruction of the upper lip after resection of a malignant melanoma. Scand J Plast Reconstr Surg Hand Surg 2005;39:45.

81. Webster RC, Coffey RJ, Kelleher RE. Total and partial reconstruction of the lower lip with innervated musclebearing flaps. Plast Reconstr Surg 1960;25:360–71.

82. Calhoun KH. Reconstruction of subtotal and total defects of the lips. In: Calhoun KH, Stiernberg CM, editors. Surgery of the lip. New York: Thieme; 1992. p. 24–34.

83. Ducic Y, Smith JE. The cervicodeltopectoral flap for single-stage resurfacing of anterolateral defects of the face and neck. Arch Facial Plast Surg 2003;5:197–201.

84. Jeng SF, Kuo YR, Wei FC, et al. Total lower lip reconstruction with a composite radial forearm-palmaris longus tendon flap: a clinical series. Plast Reconstr Surg 2004;113:19–23.

85. Ozdemir R, Ortak T, Kocer U, et al. Total lower lip reconstruction using sensate composite radial forearm flap. J Craniomaxillofac Surg 2003;14: 393–405.

86. Sadove RC, Luce EA, McGrath PC. Reconstruction of the lower lip and chin with the composite radial forearm palmaris longus free flap. Plast Reconstr Surg 1991;88:209.

87. Sakai S, Soeda S, Endo T, et al. A compound radial artery forearm flap for the reconstruction of lip and chin defect. Br J Plat Surg 1989;42:337–8.

88. Lengele BG, Testelin S, Bayet B, et al. Total lower lip functional reconstruction with a prefabricated gracilis muscle free flap. Int J Oral Maxillofac Surg 2004;33:396.

89. Chang KP, Lai CS, Tsai CC, et al. Total upper lip reconstruction with a free temporal scalp flap: long-term follow-up. Head Neck 2003;25:602.

90. Converse JM. Technique of elongation of the oral fissure and restoration of the angle of the mouth. In: Kazanjian and Converse's The Surgical Treatment of Facial Injuries. Baltimore: Williams and Wilkins; 1959. p. 795.

91. Anderson R, Kurtay M. Reconstruction of the corner of the mouth. Plast Reconstr Surg 1971;47: 463.

The Temporalis Muscle Flap and Temporoparietal Fascial Flap

Din Lam, DMD, MD[a],*, Eric R. Carlson, DMD, MD[b]

KEYWORDS

- Temporalis muscle flap • Temporoparietal fascial flap • Head and neck reconstruction
- Reconstruction • Calvarium

KEY POINTS

- The temporalis muscle (TM) flap is supplied by the anterior and posterior deep temporal arteries and innervated by a branch of the trigeminal nerve.
- The TM flap can provide both a dynamic muscle flap for facial reanimation surgery and bulky tissue for soft tissue augmentation.
- The superficial temporal artery provides the blood supply to the temporoparietal fascia (TPF).
- The thin and pliable structure of the TPF flap provides excellent tissue quality for resurfacing the ear, orbit, and the oral cavity.

INTRODUCTION

The temporal arterial system provides a favorable donor site for head and neck reconstruction and consists of the temporalis muscle (TM) flap and temporoparietal fascial (TPF) flap. These 2 flaps are based on separate vascular pedicles that permit independent flap development. Flaps developed from the temporalis system were first reported in the 1800s[1] and continue to maintain great popularity among reconstructive surgeons. Versatility in flap design by encompassing various tissue types (muscle, fascia, skin, and bone), proximity to the recipient sites, and low donor site morbidity are the primary reasons for their popular demand.

ANATOMY

The TM originates from the superior temporal line and inserts in the coronoid process of the mandible. It is covered by a thick temporalis fascia that splits into superficial and deep layers approximately 2 cm superior to the zygomatic arch. These 2 layers insert in the medial and lateral aspects of the zygomatic arch and eventually form the parotideomasseteric fascia. Between the superficial and deep fascia lies the superficial temporal fat pad. The deep temporal fat pad, an extension of the buccal fat pad, and the TM lie beneath the deep temporalis fascia (**Fig. 1**). Separating the temporalis fascia from the overlying TPF or the muscle underneath is relatively straightforward.

The TM flap has a Mathes and Nahai type III vascular pattern (2 major blood supplies). The deep temporal artery (branch of internal maxillary artery) and vein enter the medial surface of the muscle below the zygomatic arch, and the middle temporal artery (branch of superficial temporal artery) runs on the superficial surface of the muscle. The deep temporal artery divides into anterior and posterior branches: the anterior deep temporal artery (ADTA) supplies the anterior 20% of the

Disclosure: The authors have no financial disclosures to report.
[a] Department of Oral and Facial Surgery, Virginia Commonwealth University, 520 North 12th Street, Room 239, Richmond, VA 23298-0566, USA; [b] Department of Oral and Maxillofacial Surgery, University of Tennessee Medical Center, University of Tennessee Cancer Institute, 1930 Alcoa Highway, Suite 335, Knoxville, TN 37920, USA
* Corresponding author.
E-mail address: dlam@vcu.edu

Oral Maxillofacial Surg Clin N Am 26 (2014) 359–369
http://dx.doi.org/10.1016/j.coms.2014.05.004
1042-3699/14/$ – see front matter © 2014 Elsevier Inc. All rights reserved.

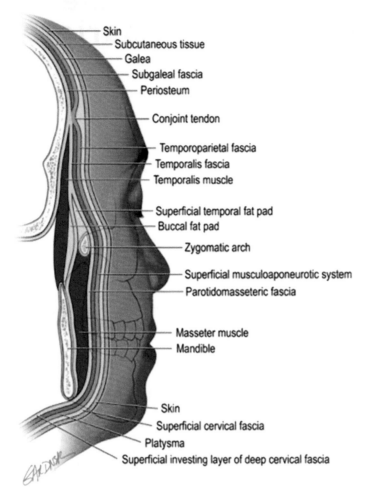

Labels on figure:
- Skin
- Subcutaneous tissue
- Galea
- Subgaleal fascia
- Periosteum
- Conjoint tendon
- Temporoparietal fascia
- Temporalis fascia
- Temporalis muscle
- Superficial temporal fat pad
- Buccal fat pad
- Zygomatic arch
- Superficial musculoaponeurotic system
- Parotidomasseteric fascia
- Masseter muscle
- Mandible
- Skin
- Superficial cervical fascia
- Platysma
- Superficial investing layer of deep cervical fascia

Fig. 1. Anatomy of fascial layers from vertex of the skull to the neck. (*Courtesy of* Dr David Webb, David Grant Medical Center, Travis Air Force Base, California.)

muscle, whereas the posterior deep temporal artery (PDTA) provides blood supply to the middle 40% of the muscle. The remaining muscle in the posterior region (40%) is supplied by the middle temporal artery.[2] The ADTA is located 2 cm anterior to the coronoid process and 2.4 cm inferior to the arch, whereas the PDTA is located 1.7 cm posterior to the coronoid process and 1.1 cm inferior to the arch.[3] Although the middle temporal artery supplies a large part of the muscle, it is commonly sacrificed during harvesting, and there is little impact on the flap's survival as a result. The function of the TM is to elevate and retract the mandible during mastication. The muscle is innervated by a branch of the trigeminal nerve, and this motor innervation must be preserved for facial reanimation surgery.

The TPF flap is a thin pliable tissue. The TPF represents the inferior extension of the galea after the temporal line and the superior extension of the subcutaneous musculoaponeurotic system

(SMAS) above the zygomatic arch. Its blood supply is derived from the superficial temporal artery in 88% of cases. Eight percent of the TPF flap is supplied by the posterior auricular artery, and the remaining 4% is supplied by the occipital artery.[4] The superficial temporal artery can be identified above the zygomatic arch and 2 cm anterior to the external auditory meatus.[5]

INDICATIONS/CONTRAINDICATIONS

The TM and TPF flaps have multiple applications for head and neck reconstruction. The TM flap provides dynamic muscular tissue, whereas the TPF flap provides thin and pliable tissue. **Table 1** lists the common indications for both flaps.

Few contraindications are associated with these flaps. Previous surgery or trauma to the scalp or temporozygomatic regions represents a contraindication for the use of these flaps. It is prudent to inform patients that there will be a significant,

Table 1 Indications for TMF and TPFF	
TMF	**TPFF**
• Reconstruction of oral defects[6–8] • Cranial base reconstruction[9–14] • Facial reanimation surgery[15,16] • Midface augmentation[17] • Obliteration of orbital defects[12]	• Reconstruction of oral defects[18,19] • Obliteration of orbital defects[20–24] • Auricular reconstruction[25–27] • Midface reconstruction with calvarial bone[28] • Reconstruction of the hair-bearing upper lip or brow[5]

visible scar in bald patients or patients with receding hairlines. Alternative flaps should also be considered in patients who have had prior radiation to the temporoparietal area, secondary to a compromised vascular supply.

PREOPERATIVE ASSESSMENT

There are few examinations required for preoperative planning of the TM and TPF flaps. A preoperative vascular assessment can be performed with a handheld Doppler or clinical palpation of the superficial temporal artery. One should also inspect for previous surgery around the scalp and auricular regions. If a functional TM flap is planned, the temporalis function should be assessed by asking the patient to clench their teeth. A bulging of the muscle in the temporal fossa should be appreciated. Temporal wasting can be a warning sign of muscle denervation. Finally, zygomatic arch integrity also needs to be assessed because an osteotomy is commonly required to assist in flap rotation.

TEMPORALIS MUSCLE FLAP TECHNIQUE
Oral Reconstruction

The patient is selected as an appropriate candidate for the TM flap primarily based on the magnitude of required oral lining as a function of the size of the defect of the maxilla (**Fig. 2**A). The patient is placed in a supine position with the head slightly turned to the side (see **Fig. 2**B). The surgical site should be prepped and draped in the usual fashion for a hemicoronal incision. The oral cavity must be prepped in a sterile fashion, and the hair is either shaved or braided preoperatively. A hemicoronal incision is marked with an inferior extension in the preauricular or endaural areas (see **Fig. 2**B). The preauricular incision should be made within 8 mm of the tragus to avoid facial nerve injury.[29] Dissection is carried out in a superior-inferior

direction in a sub-TPF plane. Raney clips are used to provide hemostasis in the scalp region. A glistening temporalis fascia in the scalp region can be easily identified (see **Fig. 2**C) and care should be taken to preserve the superficial temporal artery whenever possible. The preauricular incision should be carried down to the zygomatic arch in the subperiosteal plane. The subperiosteal dissection is carried down to expose the zygomatic arch while preserving the facial nerve. A horizontal incision is made approximately 1 cm below the temporal crest, through the temporalis fascia to expose the TM. Blunt dissection is done to separate the temporalis fascia from its muscle, and the deep temporal fat pad and middle temporal artery may be encountered. Sacrificing the middle temporal artery does not jeopardize flap survival. Blunt dissection of the TM can easily reach below the zygomatic arch. At this point, one should appreciate the medial surface of the arch that is covered by the deep layer of the temporalis fascia. Incising through the deep temporalis fascia, one can easily expose the zygomatic arch without jeopardizing the facial nerve. The zygomatic arch typically needs to be osteotomized to ease flap rotation into the recipient tissue bed such that it should be plated with a low-profile 1.2-mm titanium plate before the osteotomy (see **Fig. 2**D). When elevating the TM, an incision is made at the temporal crest through the TM to the temporal bone. A subperiosteal dissection is carefully performed to protect the vascular pedicle on the medial aspect of the flap (see **Fig. 2**E). Depending on the size of the defect, the temporalis flap can be divided into the anterior 2/3 (ADTA and PDTA) and posterior 1/3 (middle temporal artery).[2] In many cases, the anterior segment is used for reconstruction, whereas the posterior segment can be mobilized anteriorly to obliterate the temporal hollowing that will result from the rotation of the anterior portion of the muscle. Larger oral defects require the use of the entire TM for the reconstruction of oral lining. Once the flap is elevated, a tunnel is created to deliver the flap to the desired location. Reconstruction of an oral defect requires that an oral incision is made near the coronoid process. With blunt dissection of the lateral aspect of the TM, one can easily connect the infratemporal fossa dissection with that of the oral cavity. For palatal reconstruction, a bony window in the lateral sinus wall is created to connect the sinus cavity to the temporal fossa.[6] The flap is sutured to the surrounding oral mucosa to complete the reconstruction (see **Fig. 2**F). The zygomatic arch bone plate is replaced (see **Fig. 2**G) and a temporal implant is placed (see **Fig. 2**H, I) to prevent temporal hollowing. The TM

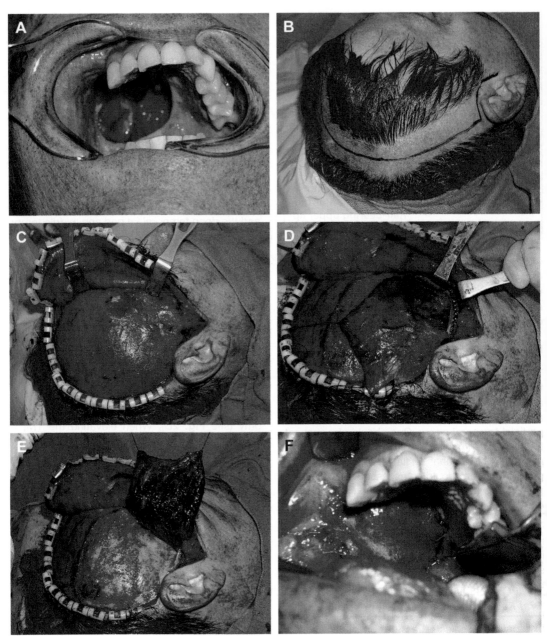

Fig. 2. An ablative defect of the oral cavity following resection of an adenoid cystic carcinoma of the right palate (*A*). The opening of the eustachian tube is noted in the lateral aspect of the defect. The size of this defect and the need for oral lining represent indications for the temporalis muscle flap with a plan for rotation of the entire muscle into the oral cavity. The access includes a hemicoronal incision (*B*). The dissection proceeds through anatomic layers including the temporoparietal fascia that results in exposure of the temporalis fascia (*C*). An incision is made through the temporalis fascia so as to protect the facial nerve. The dissection proceeds deep to the superficial layer of the temporalis fascia and inferiorly to access the zygomatic arch (*D*). A bone plate is applied to the zygomatic arch in preparation for its osteotomy. The elevation of the temporalis muscle is initiated (*E*) and the muscle is passed deep to the zygomatic arch and into the oral cavity. The muscle is sutured to the surrounding oral mucosa (*F*). The resultant defect of the temporal region is appreciated (*G*) and the bone plate is reapplied to the zygomatic arch for its anatomic alignment. A Medpor implant (*H*) is fashioned and secured to the temporal bone (*I*) to avoid temporal hollowing. The muscle surface of the flap undergoes predictable mucosalization as noted at 1 year post-operatively (*J*).

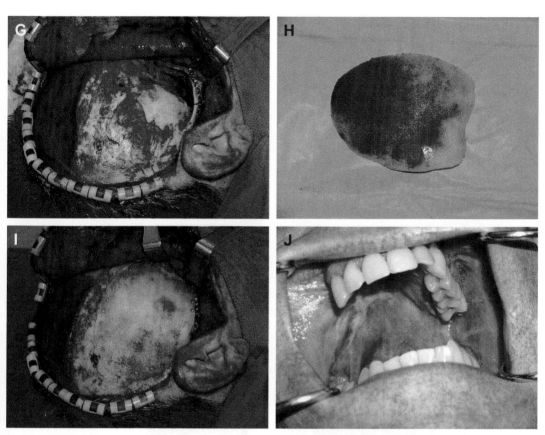

Fig. 2. (*continued*)

undergoes mucosalization over time postoperatively (see **Fig. 2**J).

Facial Reanimation Surgery

The TM flap has often been used for facial reanimation surgery. Neurorrhaphy, with or without nerve grafting, is usually indicated with acute and subacute facial nerve injury. For a paralyzed face that occurred more than 2 years previously, the TM flap is more appropriate for corner of the mouth rehabilitation. Currently, there are 2 techniques in applying the TM for facial reanimation: (1) TM flap and (2) temporalis tendon transfer.[30,31]

Conventionally, the TM flap for facial reanimation requires harvesting the middle 2 cm of the muscle. This portion of the muscle has a contraction capability of 1 to 1.5 cm and has sufficient strength to adequately mobilize the face and resist the forces of soft tissue contracture.[16] Once the flap has been elevated, transferred over the zygomatic arch, and delivered to the corner of the mouth via a subcutaneous tunnel, a 1.5-cm incision is made along both the upper and lower vermilion borders to expose the orbicularis oris muscle.[32] Mattress sutures are used to secure the TM to the lateral border of the orbicularis oris muscle. This conventional technique carries the disadvantage of distorting the contour of the lateral zygoma.

Alternatively, a temporalis tendon transfer[30,31] can be used for facial rehabilitation. Unlike the conventional technique, this is a superiorly based flap, where coronoidectomy will be performed and the muscle tendon will be detached from the coronoid process via an intra-oral incision. The detached tendon will be sutured to the modiolus near the maxillary first molar. In order for the tendon to reach to the modiolus, the posterior 2/3 of the TM must be elevated and mobilized anteriorly through the hemicoronal incision.[32] This alternative flap avoids the need for transferring the TM over the zygomatic arch and the creation of a subcutaneous tunnel.

Midfacial Augmentation

The TM flap serves as an acceptable means for midfacial soft tissue augmentation due to its muscular bulk (**Fig. 3**). The flap has a rotational radius of 8 cm^3 that allows it to reach most of the midface. If needed, the arc of rotation can be improved by removing the zygomatic arch permanently. If a full thickness defect is encountered, the

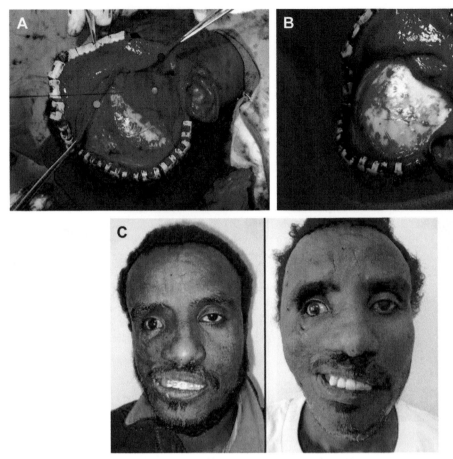

Fig. 3. Temporalis muscle flap for midfacial augmentation. Access is afforded with a hemicoronal incision with preauricular extension (*A*). (Blue circle: temporparietal flap; black circle: TM fascia; green circle: TM muscle). The TM muscle flap is transferred over the zygomatic arch to provide midface soft tissue augmentation (*B*). The preoperative (*left*) appearance of the patient is compared with the patient's post-operative appearance (*right*) (*C*).

muscle should be covered with a split thickness skin graft.

The flap is harvested as mentioned earlier and a subcutaneous tunnel is created. A 4-0 nylon suture is used to anchor the flap to the desired location. The suture is first passed through the skin at the recipient site, then through the proximal end of the temporalis, and finally through the skin inside-out near the original entry point. The suture is tied and kept in place until post-operative day 7. Depending on the size of the defect, 2 or more anchoring sutures may be required to secure the flap.

Composite Flap

The temporalis flap can incorporate the outer table of the calvarium[33] or the coronoid process[5] when the defect requires osseous reconstruction. The quality of the bone provides excellent thickness for orbital floor, maxillary wall, and palatal bone reconstruction.

COMPLICATIONS

Donor site morbidity is relatively minimal for TM flaps. This notwithstanding, some of the commonly reported complications include flap necrosis, temporal hollowing, facial nerve injury, restricted mouth opening, and hematoma or seroma formation (**Table 2**).

Table 2 TM and TPF flap complications	
TM Flap	**TPF Flap**
Flap necrosis	
Facial nerve injury	
Hematoma/seroma formation	
Temporal hollowing	Alopecia
Restricted mouth opening	

Data from Refs.[4,6,9,33]

Flap Necrosis

The TM flap is a reliable flap that realizes a failure rate of less than 2%.[9] Flap failure may be caused by inadvertent trauma to the pedicle vessel during flap development, or severe tension created within the tunnel. If excessive tension is encountered during tunnel development, one may consider decreasing the size of the flap by incorporating the anterior 1/3 of the TM flap only or removing the zygomatic arch permanently.

Temporal Hollowing

Temporal hollowing is a concern after TM flap rotation. Prevention of hollowing can be accomplished by mobilizing the posterior portion of the muscle anteriorly or using a high-density polyethylene implant (Medpor; Stryker, Kalamazoo, MI) (see **Fig. 2**H, I) to obliterate the donor site defect.[6] The posterior flap is secured at the anterior site with 3-0 Vicryl (Ethicon Inc, NJ, USA) sutures to the adjacent pericranium/temporalis fascia, and the Medpor (Stryker, Kalamazoo, MI) implant can be secured to the calvarium with a surgical wire or titanium screws (see **Fig. 2**I).

Facial Nerve Injury

Facial nerve injury is relatively uncommon in association with development of the TM flap. The incidence of transient nerve injury is approximately 10%, and permanent injury is noted in 3% of cases.[6] The temporal and zygomatic branches of the facial nerve are at greatest risk. Most injury is likely related to excessive retraction during surgery, and permanent injury is likely due to inexperience with surgical anatomy. The greatest risk of nerve injury occurs during zygomatic arch exposure. The facial nerve crosses the zygomatic arch within or beneath the TP fascia/SMAS, and it is very important to dissect in the subperiosteal plane during zygomatic dissection. Connecting the temporal region to the zygomatic region should be performed in the subtemporalis fascial plane to ensure the safety of the facial nerve.

Immediate post-operative facial nerve weakness can be managed with gentle massage and systemic oral corticosteroids for 1 week to relieve the pressure from post-operative swelling. Artificial teardrops should be prescribed to the patient for corneal protection. If no improvement has been appreciated after 6 months, surgical management should be rendered. A gold-weight implant in the upper lid is the recommended treatment option for lagophthalmos.

Restricted Mouth Opening

Initial restriction in mouth opening is likely due to post-operative edema; however, permanent restriction may be associated with the defect location in the retromolar trigone, floor of the mouth, and buccal mucosa. Clauser and colleagues[9] reported a 10% incidence rate of post-operative limited mouth opening. Although an improvement in mouth opening should be seen as the edema resolves, intense physiotherapy is recommended to restore mouth opening.

TEMPOROPARIETAL FASCIAL FLAP TECHNIQUE

Similar to the TM flap harvesting, hemicoronal and preauricular incisions are made to gain access to the TPF. The superficial temporal artery can be marked preoperatively with a handheld Doppler, and the dissection should occur within the subcutaneous plane. Unlike the temporalis fascia, the TP fascia is very adherent to the subcutaneous tissue, especially in the temporal region, which can make the dissection difficult. It is the author's recommendation to develop this plane from the inferior to superior direction for the ease of harvesting. Once the TP fascia is exposed, it is prudent to evaluate the location of the artery, and with good hemostasis, it is not uncommon to visualize the vessels embedded within the fascia. Alternatively, one can use the Doppler to trace the path of the vessel.

With the planned flap dimension decided, an incision is made central to the vessel and deep to the pericranium or temporalis fascia. Dissection is then carried down from the superior to inferior direction, elevating the TP fascia from the temporalis fascia. This elevation is relatively straightforward and avascular. As the flap advances from the temporal to zygomatic region, the surgeon must be cognizant with the anatomic location of the temporal branch of the facial nerve. The temporal branch can be traced from the tragus to a point that is 3 cm superior and 2 cm lateral to the superior orbital rim.[34]

Once the flap has been raised, a soft tissue tunnel is created to deliver the flap to the recipient tissue bed. Depending on the location of the defect, a subcutaneous tunnel is created with blunt dissection for any soft tissue augmentation or auricular reconstruction. For an intra-oral defect, an incision anterior to the masseter muscle is made through the oral mucosa and connected to the subcutaneous tunnel. Care should be taken to avoid injury to the Stensen duct. The donor site should be closed in anatomic layers over a suction drain.

Auricular Reconstruction

Auricular reconstruction using the TPF flap was first described by Nagata and colleagues[25] for congenital microtia. The TPF flap provides well-vascularized tissue for wrapping the cartilaginous framework. A split thickness skin graft is then used to cover the TPF flap. Similarly, the TPF flap can be used in cases of partial or total ear avulsion. The avulsed cartilage is separated from the overlying skin and sutured back to its original location. The TPF flap is harvested, wrapped around the cartilage, and the skin is grafted (**Fig. 4**). Ibrahim and colleagues[26] and Lin and colleagues[27] advocate this technique when microsurgical repair is not possible, and the cosmetic result is comparable to the Mladik pocket technique.[26]

Orbitomaxillary Reconstruction

Unlike the TM flap, the TPF flap does not provide the tissue bulk that is required to augment a soft tissue deficiency. However, its pliable nature serves as an excellent option to provide soft tissue lining for orbital prosthetic rehabilitation. Another indication for the TPF flap in this region is its composite flap with calvarium.[35,36] Unlike the TM flap, the parietal bone rather than temporal bone is incorporated with the flap. Harvesting the parietal bone is much safer than harvesting the temporal bone due to its increased thickness. Similar to the TM flap, the TPF composite flap provides an option for orbital floor, maxillary, and palatal osseous reconstruction.[20–24]

Oral Cavity Reconstruction

The utility of the TPF flap in oral cavity reconstruction is mostly limited to maxillary and posterior mandibular soft tissue defects (**Fig. 5**). Historically, skin grafting over the TPF flap has commonly been performed; however, Pinto and colleagues[19] reported a series of 20 cases of TPF flaps for oral mucosal reconstruction without skin grafting. Although it is not a first-line option, Parhiscar and colleagues[28] successfully reconstructed 7 mandibular and 2 palatal defects with a TPF composite flap. Most of these mandibular defects are

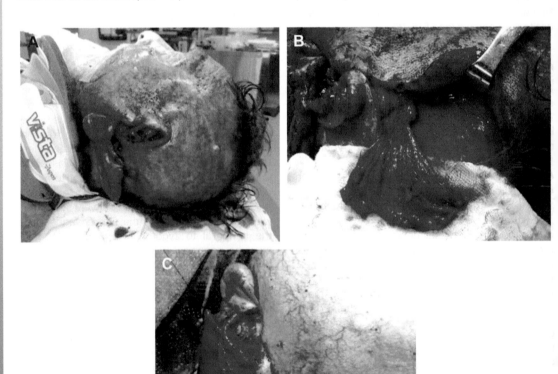

Fig. 4. (*A*) Avulsed ear; (*B*) denuding the ear cartilage and elevating the temporoparietal flap; (*C*) covering the auricular cartilage with the TPF flap.

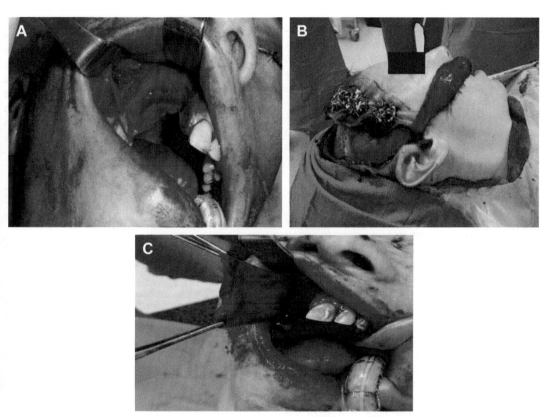

Fig. 5. Elevating the TPF flap for reconstructing oral mucosal defect. (*A*) Partial maxillectomy with overlying mucosal tissue; (*B*) elevating a temporoparietal flap; (*C*) transferring TPF flap to the recipient site.

located at the angle and posterior mandibular body, with defect sizes ranging from 4 to 5 cm.

ADDITIONAL CONSIDERATIONS
Extending Pedicle Length

When additional pedicle length is needed to reach to a distant defect, one can extend the length by

- Extending the superior margin of the flap to the midline of the scalp.
- Dissection of facial nerve and mobilization of the parotid gland.[27]

Extending the flap to the midline of the scalp carries minimal risk, whereas mobilizing the parotid gland and facial nerve may not be warranted in the author's opinion. An alternative flap should be considered in this case.

Composite Flap

The TPF flap can be raised with the underlying calvarium, which was first described by Psillakis and colleagues[35] in 1986. The parietal bone receives perforators from the superficial temporal vessel. The outer table of the parietal bone, just above the temporal line, can be harvested together with the attached TPF flap. This modification is used mostly for the reconstruction of hard tissue orbital-maxillary defects, where the thickness of the bone is relatively thin.

Endoscopically Assisted Flap Harvesting

Endoscopically assisted TPF flap development was advocated by Yano in 1999.[37] This technique has the advantages of a small surgical scar and decreased incidence of alopecia[37,38]; however, it requires more experience to safely avoid the facial nerve and vascular pedicle injuries.

COMPLICATIONS
Flap Necrosis

Park and colleagues[4] conducted a review of 109 pedicle TPF flaps and reported 5 cases of partial necrosis. This rate is comparable with that of Cheney and colleagues[39] where 3 of 21 cases developed distal flap necrosis. Most of these cases can be managed by removing the necrotic tissue and further advancing the distal portion of the flap.

Alopecia

Alopecia along the incision line is the most commonly reported complication of the TPF flap. Thermal damage during dissection or too superficial plane dissection is the most likely cause. Helling and colleagues[38] suggested that endoscopically assisted TPF flap harvesting minimizes the risk of alopecia. Management of alopecia often requires surgical removal of skin and possible advancement rotation of a scalp flap.

POST-OPERATIVE MANAGEMENT

Drains should be removed on post-operative day 2, and the patient can return to washing their hair with baby shampoo on post-operative day 3. Scalp staples or sutures should be removed on post-operative day 10.

SUMMARY

Flaps from the temporal arterial system are an excellent option for head and neck reconstruction. Advantages of these flaps include minimal donor site morbidity, relative ease of harvesting, and versatility in flap defects. These flaps are the very few head and neck regional flaps that allow the incorporation of an osseous component.

REFERENCES

1. Verneuil AA. De la creationd'une fausse articulation par sectio ou resection partielle de l'os maxillaire in- ferieure. Arch Gen Med V Serie 1872;15:284.
2. Cheung LK. The vascular anatomy of the human temporalis muscle: implications of surgical splitting techniques. Int J Oral Maxillofac Surg 1996;25:414–21.
3. Antonyshyn O, Gruss JS, Birt BD. Versatility of temporal muscle and fascial flaps. Br J Plast Surg 1988;41:118–31.
4. Park C, Lew DH, Yoo WM. An analysis of 123 temporoparietal fascial flaps: anatomic and clinical considerations in total auricular reconstruction. Plast Reconstr Surg 1999;104:1295–306.
5. Ward BB. Temporalis system in maxillary reconstruction: temporalis muscle and temporoparietal galea flaps. Atlas Oral Maxillofac Surg Clin North Am 2007;15:33–42.
6. Abubaker AO, Abouzgia MB. The temporalis muscle flap in reconstruction of intraoral defects: an appraisal of the technique. Oral Surg Oral Med Oral Pathol Oral Radiol Endod 2002;94:24–30.
7. Del Hoyo JA, Sanroman JF, Gil Diez JL, et al. The temporalis muscle flap: an evaluation and review of 38 cases. J Oral Maxillofac Surg 1994;52:143.
8. Browne JD, Holland BW. Combined intraoral and lateral temporal approach for palatal malignancies with temporalis muscle reconstruction. Arch Otolaryngol Head Neck Surg 2002;128:531–7.
9. Clauser L, Curioni C, Spanio S. The use of temporalis muscle flap in facial and craniofacial reconstructive surgery: a review of 182 cases. J Craniomaxillofac Surg 1995;23:203–14.
10. Colmenero C, Martorell V, Colmenero B, et al. Temporalis myofascial flap for maxillofacial reconstruction. J Oral Maxillofac Surg 1991;49:1067–73.
11. Chang DW, Langstein HN, Gupta A, et al. Reconstructive management of cranial base defects after tumor ablation. Plast Reconstr Surg 2001;107:1346–57.
12. Yucel A, Yazar S, Aydin Y, et al. Temporalis muscle flap for craniofacial reconstruction after tumor resection. J Craniofac Surg 2000;11(3):258–64.
13. Cordiero PG, Wolfe SA. The temporalis muscle flap revisited on its centennial advantages, newer uses, and disadvantages. Plast Reconstr Surg 1996;98:980–7.
14. McKenna MJ, Cheney ML, Borodie G, et al. Management of facial paralysis after intracranial surgery. Contemp Neural 1991;62–7.
15. Gillies HD. Experiences with fascia lata grafts in the operative treatment of facial paralysis. Proc R Soc Med 1934;27:1372–8.
16. May M, Drucker C. Temporalis muscle for facial reanimation: a 13-year experience with 224 procedures. Arch Otolaryngol Head Neck Surg 1993;119:378–82.
17. Tessier P, Tulasne JF. Surgical correction of Treacher-Collins syndrome. In: Bell WH, editor. Modern practice in orthognathic and reconstructive surgery. Philadelphia: WB Saunders; 1992. p. 1600–23.
18. Fallah DM, Baur DA, Ferguson HW, et al. Clinical application of the temporoparietal-galeal flap in closure of a chronic oronasal fistula: review of the anatomy, surgical technique, and report of a case. J Oral Maxillofac Surg 2003;61(10):1228–30.
19. Pinto FR, de Magalhaes RP, Capelli Fde A, et al. Pedicled temporoparietal galeal flap for reconstruction of intraoral defects. Ann Otol Rhinol Laryngol 2008;117:581–6.
20. Ellis DS, Toth AB, Steward WB. Temporoparietal fascial flap for orbital and eyelid reconstruction. Plast Reconstr Surg 1992;89:606–12.
21. Hanasano MM, Lee JC, Yang JS, et al. An algorithm approach to reconstructive surgery and prosthetic rehabilitation after orbital exenteration. Plast Reconstr Surg 2009;123:98–105.
22. Lai A, Cheney ML. Temporoparietal fascial flap in orbital reconstruction. Arch Otolaryngol Head Neck Surg 2000;2:196–201.
23. Kim JY, Buck DW, Johnson SA, et al. The temporoparietal fascial flap is an alternative to free flaps for

orbitomaxillary reconstruction. Plast Reconstr Surg 2010;126:880–8.

24. Spiegel JH, Varvares MA. Prevention of postexenteration complications by obliteration of the orbital cavity. Skull Base 2007;17:197–204.

25. Nagata S. A new technique of total reconstruction of the auricle for microtia. Plast Reconstr Surg 1993;92: 187–201.

26. Ibrahim SM, Zidan A, Madani S. Totally avulsed ear: new technique of immediate ear reconstruction. J Plast Reconstr Aesthet Surg 2008;61:S29–36.

27. Lin PY, Chiang YC, Hsieh CH, et al. Microsurgical replantation and salvage procedures in traumatic ear amputations. J Trauma 2010;69:E15–9.

28. Parhiscar A, Har-El G, Turk J, et al. Temporoparietal osteofascial flap for head and neck reconstruction. J Oral Maxillofac Surg 2002;60:619–22.

29. Al-kayak A, Bramley P. A modified preauricular approach to the temporomandibular joint and malar arch. Br J Oral Surg 1978;17:91–103.

30. Byrne PL, Kim M, Boahene K, et al. Temporalis tendon transfer as part of a comprehensive approach to facial reanimation. Arch Facial Plast Surg 2007;9: 234–41.

31. Labbe D, Husult M. Lengthening temporalis myoplasty and lip reanimation. Plast Reconstr Surg 2000;105:1289–97 [discussion: 1298].

32. Hadlock TA, Lindsay RW, Cheney ML. Temporalis. In: Urken ML, Cheney ML, Blackwell KE, editors. Atlas of regional and free flaps for head and neck reconstruction: flap harvest and insetting. 2nd edition. Philadelphia: Wolters Kluwer Health/Lippincott Williams & Wilkins; 2012. p. 47–58.

33. Matsuba HM, Hakki AR, Little JW, et al. The temporal fossa in head and neck reconstruction: twenty-two flaps of scalp, fascia and full thickness cranial bone. Laryngoscope 1988;98:444.

34. Seckel BR. "Facial danger zone 2." Facial danger zones: avoiding nerve injury in facial plastic surgery. 1st edition. St Louis (MO): Quality Medical Pub; 1994. p. 12–7.

35. Psillakis JM, Grotting JC, Casanova R, et al. Vascularized outer-table calvarial bone flaps. Plast Reconstr Surg 1986;78:309–17.

36. Ewers R. Reconstruction of the maxilla with a double musculoperiosteal flap in connection with a composite calvarial bone graft. Plast Reconstr Surg 1988;3: 431–6.

37. Yano H, Fukui M, Yamada K, et al. Endoscopic harvest of free temproparietal fascial flap to improve donor –site morbidity. Plast Reconstr Surg 2001; 107:1003–9.

38. Helling ER, Okoro S, Kim G, et al. Endoscope-assisted temporoparietal fascia harvest for auricular reconstruction. Plast Reconstr Surg 2008;121: 1598–605.

39. Cheney ML, Varvares MA, Nadol JB. The temporoparietal fascial flap in head and neck reconstruction. Arch Otolaryngol Head Neck Surg 1993;119: 618–23.

Submental Island Flap

Allen Cheng, DDS, MD[a,b,c], Tuan Bui, MD, DMD[a,b,c,d],*

KEYWORDS

- Submental • Flap • Local • Island

KEY POINTS

- The submental island flap is based off of the submental artery, which branches from the facial artery along the superior side of the submandibular gland; its venae comitantes, which drain into the facial vein; and the submental vein, which drains into the common facial vein.
- The submental island flap matches the facial skin well.
- The size of the skin paddle is limited by cervical laxity.
- The skin perforators are variable, and they can be protected by including both the anterior belly of the digastric and the mylohyoid muscles with the flap.
- The standard design allows for reconstruction of defects of lower region of face, floor of mouth defects, and oral tongue defects.
- The reach of this flap can be extended by using reverse flow patterns.
- Elective tracheostomies should be performed after neck closure rather than at the beginning of the surgery.
- Complete clearance of Level I nodes is difficult when using a submental island flap.

INTRODUCTION

Reconstruction of soft tissue defects of the oral cavity and face is a complex undertaking. Several flaps are available, each with their advantages and drawbacks. These flaps include local and regional axial patterned flaps, random patterned flaps, and free flaps. Local flaps raised using cervical skin are particularly helpful for facial soft tissue defects. These flaps provide good matching for skin color and thickness. However, they do have limitations, including unpredictable viability and limited mobility.

The submental island flap is a useful addition to the reconstructive surgeon's armamentarium. Initially described in 1993 by Martin and colleagues,[1] modifications of its design allow for it to achieve wide mobility, good predictability, and excellent skin color match. The donor site scar is

well hidden in the shadow of the mandible. This flap also has the advantage of tightening cutis laxia of the submental skin. There is decreased operating room time and length of hospital stay associated with reconstructing defects with a submental island flap when compared with the radial forearm free flap.[2] In addition, the flap has broad indications, having been adapted for reconstruction of defects of the pharynx, larynx, and proximal esophagus.[3–5]

This article discusses the uses of this versatile flap, the surgical technique for raising this flap, some precautions to be taken when using this flap, and the postoperative care.

FLAP SPECIFICATIONS

Type of flap: fasciocutaneous, myocutaneous, or osteomyocutaneous; Mathes and Nahai

[a] Department of Oral, Head and Neck Oncology, Providence Portland Cancer Center, 819 Northeast 47th Avenue, Portland, OR 97213, USA; [b] Oral and Maxillofacial Surgery, Legacy Emanuel Medical Center, 2801 North Gantenbein Avenue, Portland, OR 97227, USA; [c] Department of Oral and Maxillofacial Surgery, Oregon Health Sciences University, 611 Southwest Campus Drive, Portland, OR 97201, USA; [d] Head and Neck Surgical Associates, 1849 Northwest Kearney Street, Suite 300, Portland, OR 97209, USA
* Corresponding author. Head and Neck Surgical Associates, 1849 Northwest Kearney Street, Suite 300, Portland, OR 97209.
E-mail address: tgbui@hnsa1.com

Oral Maxillofacial Surg Clin N Am 26 (2014) 371–379
http://dx.doi.org/10.1016/j.coms.2014.05.005
1042-3699/14/$ – see front matter © 2014 Elsevier Inc. All rights reserved.

classification: Type   C   (myocutaneous perforator)

Skin paddle size: 7 × 15 cm

Artery: submental artery, 5 cm length, 1.5 mm diameter

Vein: small venae comitantes, which drain into facial vein (2.5 mm); and submental vein that drains separately into the common facial vein (3 mm)

Muscle: harvested with platysma, ipsilateral anterior belly of the digastric (optional), and a portion of the mylohyoid (optional)

ANATOMY

The submental island flap is a fasciocutaneous flap that includes a rhomboid area of skin, subcutaneous tissue, and platysma located below the inferior border of the mandible. Injection studies into the submental artery have found that it can supply a large skin paddle, as great as 10 × 16 cm, reaching from one angle of the mandible to the contralateral angle.[6] Although this horizontal dimension includes an area supplied by bilateral submental arteries, the entire flap can be perfused by one side. Practically speaking, the anteroposterior dimension of the skin flap that can be harvested is limited by the ability to achieve primary closure, which depends on the patient's skin laxity, which can be estimated by marking out the desired anteroposterior dimension of the flap and attempting to pinch the marks together with forceps. A 6- to 8-cm anteroposterior dimension is usually attainable.

As mentioned above, the flap is supplied by the submental artery. The submental artery is a branch of the facial artery. Venous drainage is based on venae comitantes that drain into the facial vein as well as the submental vein.

The submental artery branches off of the facial artery anterior to the submandibular gland. The facial artery courses anteriorly, superficial to the surface of the submandibular gland and then along the undersurface of the mylohyoid muscle. A third of the time, the artery may run between the submandibular gland and inferior border of the mandible.[7] Occasionally, the artery may follow an intraglandular path. The submental artery runs deep to the anterior belly of the digastric muscle 70% to 80% of the time.[6,7]

The submental artery supplies branches to the lower lip, the mylohyoid muscle, the digastric muscle, the mandibular periosteum, the platysma, and the submental skin. The locations of the perforator vessels connecting the submental artery to the subdermal plexus (which perfuses the areas listed above) are variable. There may

be a single perforator, 2 perforators on either side of the digastric muscle, or multiple perforators from the digastric muscle.[7] It is, therefore, essential to include this wide area with the flap to be sure that the perforators remain with the harvested flap. These perforators can be protected by including the ipsilateral anterior belly of the digastric muscle as well as a cuff of mylohyoid muscle.[8] This technique does not result in a significant functional deficit and is preferred by the authors.

There are 2 nerves within the region of this dissection. The marginal mandibular branch of the facial nerve follows a course within the superficial layer of deep cervical fascia that overlies the submandibular gland. The motor nerve to the mylohyoid muscle follows a path deep to the submental artery.

USES OF THE SUBMENTAL ISLAND FLAP

- Soft tissue defects of the lower part of face.
- Soft tissue defects of the midface and upper region of face, which may require
  - Division of the facial artery distal to the submental artery take off and division of the facial vein with venous anastomosis near the recipient site (superficial temporal vein),
  - Division of the facial artery and vein proximal to the submental artery, based on retrograde flow, or
  - Division of the facial artery proximal to the submental artery and facial vein proximal and distal with anastomosis near the recipient site.
- Malar augmentation with fascia flap only.[9,10]
- Reconstruction of defects with hair-bearing skin.[11]
- Tongue and/or floor of mouth defects.
- Buccal mucosa defects.
- Palatal defects.[12]
- Nasal reconstruction.[13]
- Lip reconstruction.[14–16]
- Cervical esophagus repair or reconstruction.[3,17,18]
- Repair of hemilaryngectomy defects.[5]
- Reconstruction of neopharynx after total laryngectomy.
- Repair of pharyngocutaneous fistulas.[4]
- Coverage of hardware used in spine surgery.[19]

CONTRAINDICATIONS

There are few absolute contraindications to using the submental island flap for head and neck reconstruction. The first is severe medical comorbidities that preclude major surgery. The second is regional metastatic disease involving the ipsilateral Level I lymphatic tissue bed. This condition would make it extremely difficult to raise the flap and preserve the pedicle while maintaining an oncologically sound neck dissection.

In addition, caution should be exercised when choosing this flap in certain situations. Similar to the patients with a Level I node-positive neck, in the patients with head and neck cancer with a node-negative neck, a positive node outside of Level I, or a deeply invasive floor of mouth tumor the surgeon needs to meticulously inspect the node-bearing tissue that is raised as part of the flap. A good portion of the fibroadipose lymphatic tissue raised with the flap can and should be safely removed and included with the neck dissection specimen. Hayden and colleagues[20] found no tumor recurrences in his case series of 50 patients with oral squamous cell carcinoma without nodal metastases in the Level I basin and whose defects were reconstructed with submental island flaps. However, it is technically difficult to remove all the node-bearing tissue from under the flap, so if the patient is at high risk for metastasis to this region, an alternative flap should be considered. The authors prefer to not use this flap in patients with a node-positive neck or deeply invasive floor of mouth tumor.

Local trauma, particularly burns, causes a regional zone of injury where there is microscopic endothelial damage that increases risk of flap failure. For traumatic defects, care should be taken when selecting the submental island flap if the pedicle is adjacent to the site of injury.

As mentioned above, primary closure of the donor site defect requires neck skin laxity. Before raising the flap, the surgeon should determine whether the planned width could be closed primarily. If not, an alternative flap should be considered.

PREOPERATIVE CONSIDERATIONS

Preoperative evaluation is the same as in any other patient undergoing head and neck surgery. No special precautions need to be taken in patients with a history concerning for hypercoagulability, unless one is planning on using a modification that requires vessel anastomosis. In that case, a hypercoagulable panel should be ordered. Although sufficient evidence-based guidelines are not available, in this setting the authors use systemic heparin intraoperatively just before anastomosis followed by therapeutic heparin for 72 hours.

PROCEDURE
Patient Preparation and Positioning

Patient should be placed in supine position. A shoulder roll or an adjustable Mayfield headrest is used to place the neck in slight extension. Bed is tilted into a slight reverse Trendelenburg position for the ease of flap harvesting.

The patient should be prepared and draped in the standard manner for head and neck procedures, exposing the patient from above the defect superiorly to just below the clavicles inferiorly.

No invasive monitoring is absolutely required, unless indicated by the patient's comorbidities.

Surgical Technique

Step 1: identify the location of perforator vessels using a Doppler
This step is especially critical when the size of the skin paddle is small, because there is the opportunity to inadvertently exclude the perforator from the elevated flap.

Step 2: plan the skin flap
Measure the size of the defect (**Figs. 1** and **2**). Appropriately sized skin paddle can be marked out in the submental region. Place the superior incision behind and below the inferior border of the mandible to adequately hide the scar. The skin paddle is a crescent-shaped ellipse centered at the midline with the anteroposterior axis perpendicular to the patient's midsagittal plane (**Fig. 3**). However, this can be modified where the skin paddle is more to one side and the horizontal axis of the ellipse is obliquely oriented and along a line suited for a neck dissection incision, such that when this paddle is included with a neck dissection, closure can be performed without an irregular

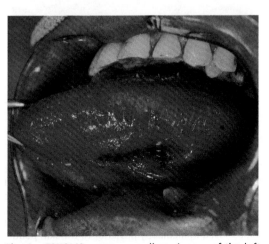

Fig. 1. cT2N0M0 squamous cell carcinoma of the left lateral region of tongue.

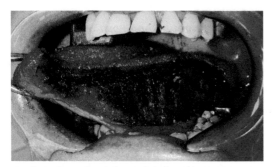

Fig. 2. Defect after left partial glossectomy.

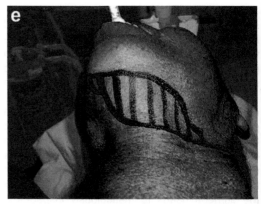

Fig. 4. Modification of skin paddle placement to allow for primary closure without a tricone deformity. (*From* Varghese BT. Optimal design of a submental artery island flap. J Plast Reconstr Aesthet Surg 2011;64:e183–4; with permission.)

incision and large tricone deformities (**Fig. 4**).[21] Alternatively, plan the incision with a Burow triangle (see **Fig. 3**).

The inferior incision's design is based on the needs of the defect to be reconstructed. However, the maximum anteroposterior dimension is limited by the ability to achieve primary closure, which is determined by the amount of laxity in the neck skin. Once the desired anteroposterior width of the flap is marked out, pinch the skin between the incisions to gauge whether it is feasible to obtain primary closure. A history of prior

radiotherapy also limits skin laxity and the ability of the wound to heal under tension. If the skin is not lax enough, reduce the width or select another flap.

Design the skin paddle to include the perforators identified in Step 1. Because the locations of the perforators are variable, designing smaller skin flaps is limited by the need to place them in such a way as to incorporate the perforator. At a minimum, the skin paddle must include an area overlying the anterior belly of the ipsilateral digastric muscle and a short distance medial and lateral to it. It may be preferable to design a larger skin paddle and then de-epithelialize the excess skin.

Step 3: make inferior incision and elevate subplatysmal skin flaps to expose up to the digastric tendon

Make an incision along the planned inferior aspect of the skin paddle, extending into a planned cervical incision if a neck dissection is to be done as well. If the inferior incision is below the hyoid bone, elevate the skin paddle superiorly in a broad front in a subplatysmal plane. Raise the skin paddle up to the level of the hyoid bone. Dissect and identify the intermediate tendon of the digastric muscle at its attachment to the hyoid bone. Elevate the inferior skin flap as needs dictate for the planned surgery.

If the inferior extent of the skin paddle is above the hyoid bone, take the incision down to the depth of the superficial layer of the deep cervical fascia. Raise the inferior skin flap below the level of the hyoid bone or lower as needs dictate for the planned surgery. As mentioned above, dissect out and identify the intermediate tendon of the digastric muscle.

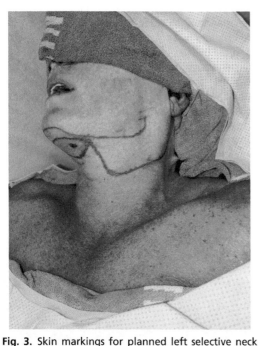

Fig. 3. Skin markings for planned left selective neck dissection along with elevation of submental island flap for reconstruction. The blue dot represents the location of skin perforators from the submental artery identified with a Doppler probe. A Burow triangle will be removed immediately posterior to the skin paddle to allow for the wound closure into a curvilinear incision without any cone deformities.

Step 4: identify vascular pedicle in submandibular triangle

As the incision is carried laterally, the common facial vein is observed crossing superficial to the posterior belly of the digastric muscle. This vein should be dissected out and protected.

Identify the submandibular gland within the submandibular triangle. In some patients, the gland is ptotic and may lie just below the digastric tendon. Use blunt dissection to enter the capsule that envelops the gland. Begin to raise the superior flap in a plane just above the gland and deep to the superficial layer of deep cervical fascia. As the dissection proceeds along the gland, several branches of the facial artery are encountered. Follow these until the facial artery is identified running along its intraglandular course. Dissect the artery superiorly until the submental artery is found branching anteriorly along the superior aspect of the gland. Once the submental artery is identified, dissect it out anteriorly until it reaches the posterior free border of the mylohyoid muscle.

Removal of the submandibular gland can be helpful during this dissection and may be necessary if skeletonization of the pedicle is required to lengthen the axis of rotation of the flap.

Step 5: make superior incision and identify the facial vessels and marginal mandibular nerve

Make the superior incision. Starting medially, take the incision down to and through platysma. Identify the anterior belly of the digastric muscle as it attaches to the lingual aspect of the anterior mandible. Carefully extend the dissection laterally. Identify the facial artery and vein as they cross the inferior border of the mandible near the antegonial notch. In the standard design for the submental island flap based on anterograde flow, these vessels may be ligated and divided after the submental artery has been identified. Doing so increases the length of the pedicle by 1 to 2 cm. During this dissection, it is essential to identify the marginal mandibular branch of the facial nerve and protect it. This branch may be most easily found as it crosses superficial to the facial vein. Use of a nerve stimulator can aid in locating this nerve.

Step 6: begin elevating the skin paddle from distal to proximal

Starting at the portion of the skin paddle most distal from the pedicle, begin elevating the skin paddle in a plane superficial to the mylohyoid muscle. If the skin paddle crosses the midline, the portion that is contralateral to the midline may be elevated in a subplatysmal plane. Continue raising the flap until the ipsilateral anterior belly of the digastric muscle is encountered. Take care to avoid injuring any perforators that may run medial to the anterior belly of the digastric to supply the subdermal plexus of the skin paddle.

Step 7: divide the attachments of the anterior belly of the digastric muscle

Divide the anterior belly of the digastric muscle at its attachment to the mandible and at the intermediate tendon.

The authors prefer a modification proposed by Patel and colleagues,[8] which includes a cuff of mylohyoid muscle with the flap to add an additional layer of protection for the submental artery and its perforators. At the medial border of the anterior belly of the digastric muscle, dissect through the mylohyoid muscle to the underlying geniohyoid muscle. Divide the attachments of the mylohyoid from the mandible above and the hyoid below. This process obviates the need to identify and protect the perforators while elevating the deep portion of the flap. However, this should be performed with caution if there is considerable risk of tumor extension or metastasis into Level I.

Step 8: complete elevation of the flap from distal

Once the anterior belly of the digastric and mylohyoid attachments have been divided, continue using blunt dissection to elevate the mylohyoid muscle off of the underlying geniohyoid, working toward the submental artery pedicle (**Fig. 5**). If a portion of the skin paddle extends lateral to the pedicle, elevate this in a subplatysmal plane until it joins with the prior dissection.

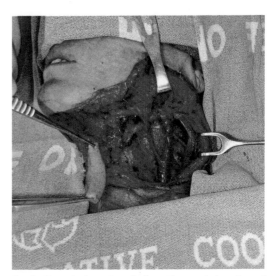

Fig. 5. Completion of neck dissection and elevation of the submental island flap. The ipsilateral anterior belly of the digastric muscle and a portion of the mylohyoid muscle are included with the flap.

Step 9: create a tunnel

Use blunt dissection to create a subcutaneous tunnel to the desired defect. Ensure that the tunnel allows easy passage of 3 fingers to avoid compression on the pedicle. Transfer the flap intraorally, taking care not to twist the island around the axis of the pedicle (**Fig. 6**). Suture the elevated flap to the edges of the defect (**Fig. 7**).

Step 10: closure

Drape the cervical skin flaps together. It may be necessary to excise excess skin to obtain a closure that is free of tricone deformities (**Fig. 8**). If an inferior cervical skin flap was not developed, do so now to allow for tension-free closure. Avoid undermining the superior cervical skin flap over the mandible and mentum, because this can lead to lower lip eversion.

At the midline, place several deep sutures to approximate the cervical skin flaps down to the hyoid periosteum. This process helps in preserving definition at the cervicomental angle. Then close the wound in layers. The authors typically place a suction drain in the wound before closure.

Step 11: tracheostomy, if indicated

If a considerable amount of prolonged airway swelling is anticipated with associated risk of airway compromise, consider performing a tracheostomy. A surgical airway is advisable if using

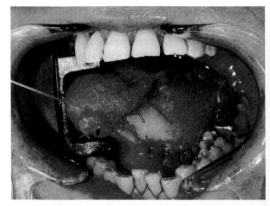

Fig. 7. The skin paddle is sutured in place. Care is taken not to twist the flap along the axis of the pedicle.

the submental flap for tongue or floor of mouth reconstructions.

If a tracheostomy is indicated and planned, it is preferable to perform this at the end of the operation, rather than at the beginning of the surgery. If a tracheostomy is performed at the onset of the operation rather then at the time of closure, undermining the inferior skin flap and pulling it superiorly to close the submental donor site defect has the effect of moving the transcutaneous tunnel for the tracheostomy superiorly, away from the opening in the trachea. Although not immediately apparent, this can greatly complicate tracheostomy tube changes or replacement of the tracheostomy tube if it is inadvertently dislodged.

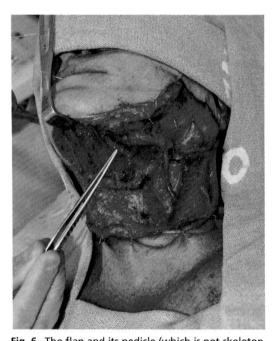

Fig. 6. The flap and its pedicle (which is not skeletonized) are passed through a tunnel into the floor of mouth.

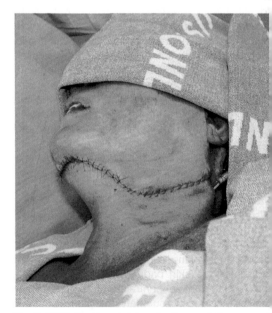

Fig. 8. With the Burow triangle removed, the wounds are closed into a curvilinear incision.

VARIATIONS IN TECHNIQUE

There are several variations in flap design to allow for extension of the length of the flap for use in defects as superior as the temporal region or as far posterior as the occiput. In addition, once the anatomy is understood, the flap may be elevated from any direction as the appropriate landmarks are identified. The authors find the technique described above to be the simplest way to raise the flap.

Reverse Flow Venous Drainage via the External Jugular Vein

The first limitation in lengthening the pedicle is tethering of the common facial vein to the internal jugular vein. Martin and colleagues[22] described a variation in the technique that they initially described by using reverse flow drainage to the external jugular vein. In this schema, the common facial vein is divided. Venous blood then follows a reverse flow pattern along the anterior branch of the retromandibular vein, and then back down the posterior communicating branch into the external jugular vein.

This technique increases the length of the pedicle by up to 5 cm. However, anatomic variations exist where either the posterior branch of the retromandibular vein is missing or a valve in the anterior branch prevents reverse flow. In these situations, an alternative technique should be sought.

Retrograde Flow Artery and Reverse Flow Venous Drainage

Alternatively, both the facial artery and common facial vein are divided proximal to the takeoffs of the submental artery and vein (**Fig. 9**). Venous drainage is also reverse flow via the angular vein. The marginal mandibular nerve is skeletonized anteriorly and posteriorly to allow for the flap to be passed underneath. Otherwise, the nerve would tether the pedicle at their intersection, limiting the full arc of rotation.

There have been reports of issues with venous congestion as well as total flap loss using this technique, presumably from valves within the common facial vein.[23]

Hybrid Flap

Sterne and colleagues[23] described a hybrid flap, with the submental artery remaining pedicled to the facial artery based on retrograde flow and the vein anastomosed to a donor vein in closer proximity to the defect. This flap increases the length of the pedicle by more than 5 cm and is

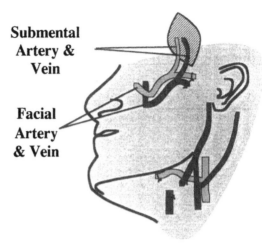

Fig. 9. Schema using reverse arterial flow and venous drainage via the angular artery and vein. (*From* Sterne GD, Januszkiewicz JS, Hall PN, et al. The submental island flap. Br J Plast Surg 1996;49:85–9; with permission.)

also feasible when reverse venous flow to the external jugular vein is not feasible because of either the absence of the posterior communicating branch of the retromandibular vein or the presence of a valve within the anterior communicating branch of the retromandibular vein.

In this schema, the facial artery is divided proximal to the submental artery takeoff. A vein in proximity to the defect is identified. The vein is divided as proximal as allowable, which preserves standard drainage from the anticipated recipient vein. For example, if the recipient vein is the facial or superficial temporal vein, the venous pedicle is divided at the submental vein just distal to its takeoff from the facial vein. If the external jugular vein is to be used as recipient vessel, the pedicle can be divided at the common facial vein distal to its takeoff from the internal jugular vein. The venous pedicle is than anastomosed to the recipient vein (**Fig. 10**).

If this is to be done in conjunction with a neck dissection, the neck dissection should be completed before division of the venous pedicle.

Free Flap

The submental island flap can also be used as a free flap by performing microvascular anastomoses of both the arteries and veins.

POSTOPERATIVE CARE

Much of the postoperative care is similar to that provided for most patients undergoing head and neck surgery. Drains are kept on suction and meticulously stripped in the immediate

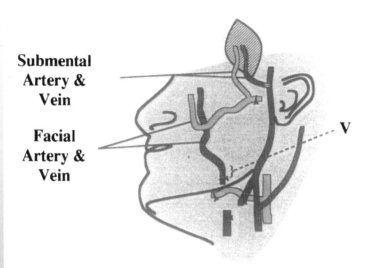

**Submental
Artery &
Vein**

**Facial
Artery &
Vein**

Fig. 10. Schema using a hybrid flap combining reverse arterial flow with a venous anastomosis in proximity to the defect. (*From* Sterne GD, Januszkiewicz JS, Hall PN, et al. The submental island flap. Br J Plast Surg 1996;49:85–9; with permission.)

postoperative period to avoid hematoma formation. The head of bed is kept elevated to reduce swelling. Because the neck is closed under tension, excessive neck extension should be prohibited. The patient should be maintained in a neutral head position or with slight neck flexion.

If a standard anterograde flap design is used, flap monitoring is unnecessary. The authors do not routinely use antiplatelets or anticoagulants for their pedicled flaps. If a reverse flow, hybrid, or free flap design is used, then flap monitoring should be performed based on the surgeon's institution's standards.

COMPLICATIONS

- Flap failure
- Hematoma
- Infection
- Wound dehiscence
- Injury of marginal mandibular branch of facial nerve
- Incomplete neck dissection of Level I

FUTURE CONSIDERATIONS

The submental island flap is relatively new in its description. Although it is more commonly used for lower facial defects as well as floor of mouth and tongue defects, new applications for this versatile flap continue to be developed, many of which are outlined above. Several surgeons have creatively used this flap in combination with other flaps to reconstruct complex composite defects of the face. Because use breeds familiarity, more indications for this versatile flap may emerge.

SUMMARY

The submental island flap is a versatile flap that, when creatively used, has broad applications for facial reconstruction. This flap has a dependable blood supply and can be raised easily, and its skin matches well with facial skin. The limitations of this flap include need for cervical skin laxity, difficulty with comprehensive clearance of level I nodal tissue, and the length of its pedicle. This flap should be included as part of every facial reconstructive surgeon's armamentarium.

REFERENCES

1. Martin D, Baudet J, Mondie JM, et al. The submental island skin flap. A surgical protocol. Prospects of use. Ann Chir Plast Esthet 1990;35:480–4 [in French].
2. Paydarfar JA, Patel UA. Submental island pedicled flap vs radial forearm free flap for oral reconstruction: comparison of outcomes. Arch Otolaryngol Head Neck Surg 2011;137:82–7.
3. Janssen DA, Thimsen DA. The extended submental island lip flap: an alternative for esophageal repair. Plast Reconstr Surg 1998;102:835–8.
4. Demir Z, Velidedeoglu H, Çelebioglu S. Repair of pharyngocutaneous fistulas with the submental artery island flap. Plast Reconstr Surg 2005;115:38–44.
5. Vural E, Suen JY. The submental island flap in head and neck reconstruction. Head Neck 2013;22:572–8.
6. Faltaous AA, Yetman RJ. The submental artery flap: an anatomic study. Plast Reconstr Surg 1996;97:56–60 [discussion: 61–2].

7. Magden O, Edizer M, Tayfur V, et al. Anatomic study of the vasculature of the submental artery flap. Plast Reconstr Surg 2004;114:1719–23.

8. Patel UA, Bayles SW, Hayden RE. The submental flap: a modified technique for resident training. Laryngoscope 2007;117:186–9.

9. Chen WL, Yang ZH, Huang ZQ, et al. Facial contour reconstruction after benign tumor ablation using reverse facial-submental artery deepithelialized submental island flaps. J Craniofac Surg 2010;21: 83–6.

10. Tan O, Atik B, Parmaksizoglu D. Soft-tissue augmentation of the middle and lower face using the deep-ithelialized submental flap. Plast Reconstr Surg 2007;119:873–9.

11. Demir Z, Kurtay A, Sahin U, et al. Hair-bearing submental artery island flap for reconstruction of mustache and beard. Plast Reconstr Surg 2003; 112:423–9.

12. Genden EM, Buchbinder D, Urken ML. The submental island flap for palatal reconstruction: a novel technique. J Oral Maxillofac Surg 2004;62:387–90.

13. Tan O, Kiroglu AF, Atik B, et al. Reconstruction of the columella using the prefabricated reverse flow submental flap: a case report. Head Neck 2006; 28:653–7.

14. Kitazawa T, Harashina T, Taira H, et al. Bipedicled submental island flap for upper lip reconstruction. Ann Plast Surg 1999;42:83–6.

15. Koshima I, Inagawa K, Urushibara K, et al. Combined submental flap with toe web for reconstruction of the lip with oral commissure. Br J Plast Surg 2000; 53:616–9.

16. Yilmaz M, Menderes A, Barutçu A. Submental artery island flap for reconstruction of the lower and mid face. Ann Plast Surg 1997;39:30–5.

17. Zhang B, Wang JG, Chen WL, et al. Reverse facial-submental artery island flap for reconstruction of oropharyngeal defects following middle and advanced-stage carcinoma ablation. Br J Oral Maxillofac Surg 2011;49:194–7.

18. Wang WH, Hwang TZ, Chang CH, et al. Reconstruction of pharyngeal defects with a submental island flap after hypopharyngeal carcinoma ablation. ORL J Otorhinolaryngol Relat Spec 2012;74:304–9.

19. Abboud O, Shedid D, Ayad T. Reconstruction of the prevertebral space with a submental flap: a novel application. J Plast Reconstr Aesthet Surg 2013; 66(12):1763–5.

20. Howard BE, Nagel TH, Donald CB, et al. Oncologic safety of the submental flap for reconstruction in oral cavity malignancies. Otolaryngol Head Neck Surg 2013;149(2 Suppl):40.

21. Varghese BT. Optimal design of a submental artery island flap. J Plast Reconstr Aesthet Surg 2011;64: e183–4.

22. Martin D, Legaillard P, Bakhach J, et al. Reverse flow YV pedicle extension: a method of doubling the arc of rotation of a flap under certain conditions. Ann Chir Plast Esthet 1994;39:403–14 [in French].

23. Sterne GD, Januszkiewicz JS, Hall PN, et al. The submental island flap. Br J Plast Surg 1996;49:85–9.

The Platysma Myocutaneous Flap

Dale A. Baur, DDS, MD[a],*, Jonathan Williams, DMD, MD[a], Xena Alakaily, DDS[b]

KEYWORDS

- Reconstruction • Platysma flap • Local flap • Defects of oral cavity

KEY POINTS

- The platysma myocutaneous flap is a reliable and versatile tool of head and neck reconstruction.
- The platysma myocutaneous flap includes good color match, easy access to the donor site in the same operative field, minimal donor site morbidity, ease in closing the donor site primarily, and appropriate flap thickness for most oral or facial defects.
- Use of this flap results in minimal contour and mobility changes of the neck.
- Defects of the oral cavity in the range of 50 to 75 cm^2 can be reconstructed with the platysma myocutaneous flap.

Reconstructing defects of the oral mucosa or skin of the lower one-third of the face can be accomplished by a variety of techniques. Presented herein are two versions of the platysma myocutaneous flap, which is a reliable, axial pattern, pedicled flap capable of providing excellent one-stage reconstruction of such defects. Also included is a review of other uses of this flap in head and neck surgery. The advantages of the platysma flap include good color match, easy access to the donor site in the same operative field, minimal donor site morbidity, ease in closing the donor site primarily, and appropriate flap thickness for most oral or facial defects.[1] In general, defects of the oral cavity in the range of 50 to 75 cm^2 can be reconstructed with the platysma myocutaneous flap.[2] Use of this flap results in minimal contour and mobility changes of the neck. Donor site scarring is minimal and well accepted. The platysma flap can be used reliably even when an ipsilateral neck dissection is performed, as long as the surgeon takes care to preserve the vascular pedicle during the dissection. When compared with the radial forearm microvascular free flap, the platysma flap has a better color match, can be harvested in much less time, and has significantly less donor site morbidity.[3] When compared with the pectoralis major myocutaneous flap, the platysma flap is less bulky, has a better color match to facial skin, and is faster and easier to harvest with less morbidity.

Based on the dominant blood supply, there are three different variations of the platysma flap. The inferiorly based flap, with an arterial supply from the transverse cervical artery, has no application in oral and facial reconstruction.[3] As discussed herein, the superiorly based and posteriorly based versions of the flap have wide application in the oral and facial region. In addition to their use in reconstructing oral and facial extirpative defects, these flaps can be used for reconstruction of the lip, ear, pharynx, and trachea. Other uses include hypopharygeal strictures and additional tissue bulk for mild cases of facial hypoplasia. Contraindications to using these flaps include previous radiation treatment to the neck and previous surgical procedures to the neck in which the dominant blood supply has been violated or the muscle previously transected.

No financial disclosures for any of the authors.
[a] Department of Oral and Maxillofacial Surgery, University Hospitals of Cleveland, Case Western Reserve University, 2124 Cornell Road, Cleveland, OH 44106–4905, USA; [b] Department of Oral and Maxillofacial Surgery, Case Western Reserve University, 2124 Cornell Road, Cleveland, OH 44106–4905, USA
* Corresponding author.
E-mail address: Dale.baur@case.edu

oralmaxsurgery.theclinics.com

ANATOMY

The awake patient can actively demonstrate the anatomy and extent of the platysma muscle by lifting the chin and grimacing. The thin, quadrangular-shaped, paired platysma muscles (**Fig. 1**) lie in the superficial fascia of the neck.[4] They are derived from second brachial arch. The muscle originates from the superficial fascia of the pectoral and deltoid muscles, coursing obliquely over the clavicle to its insertion at the corner of the mouth and inferior part of the cheek.[5] It is absent in the midline of the neck and the superior portion of the posterior triangle. Immediately deep to the platysma is the superficial layer of the deep cervical fascia. Fibers of the platysma insert with the angle of the mandible and depressor muscles of the lip and chin. The anterior fibers decussate over the chin with the contralateral platysma. When the muscle contracts, it pulls the corner of the mouth inferiorly and laterally, partially contributing to mouth opening.[3]

The submental branch of the facial artery provides arterial blood superiorly. The submental artery is the largest branch of the facial artery providing the most plentiful blood supply to a superiorly based flap.[5] Branches of the transverse cervical artery supply the platysma muscle inferiorly. From the posterior triangle of the neck, the muscle receives branches from the occipital and posterior auricular arteries. The superior thyroid artery perfuses the muscle from the anterior triangle of the neck.[5] Fasciocutaneous arterial perforators from the muscle itself supply the overlying skin. At the posterior extent of the muscle lies the external jugular vein, providing for venous drainage. The anterior jugular veins, the submental vein, and the anterior communicating veins also contribute to venous drainage.[3] Innervation of the platysma muscle is from the cervical branch of the seventh cranial nerve. These branches are generally multiple and enter the muscle on the deep surface from a superior direction in the

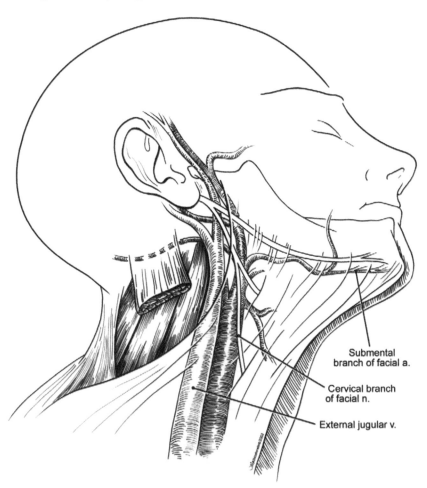

Submental branch of facial a.

Cervical branch of facial n.

External jugular v.

Fig. 1. Diagram of the platysma muscle with associated structures. (*From* Baur DA. The plastysma myocutaneous flap. Oral Maxillofac Clin North Am 2003;15(4):559–64.)

area of the angle of the mandible and sternocleido-mastoid muscle.[6] At times, the cervical branch can be maintained to provide an innervated muscle flap for facial reanimation. The marginal mandibular branch of the facial nerve is also found deep to the platysma, usually at or near the inferior border of the mandible. Cutaneous sensation of the anterolateral neck is supplied by the transverse cervical nerves (C2, C3, C4), found curving around the lateral mid sternocleidomastoid muscle.

POSTERIORLY BASED PLATYSMA FLAP

The posteriorly based platysma flap receives its axial blood supply primarily from branches of the occipital artery, which are located within the fascia at the anterior border of the sternocleidomastoid muscle. Collateral circulation from the superior

thyroid and posterior auricular arteries may also contribute.[7] Venous drainage for this flap is through the external jugular vein. For this reason, one must maintain the integrity of the external jugular vein at the base of the flap to minimize venous congestion and improve flap survival.[3] The external jugular vein may be ligated superiorly if necessary. In this version of the platysma flap, it is not possible to maintain the cervical branch of the facial nerve. Wide exposure of the muscle is important to assess and measure the arc of rotation into the surgical defect.[3] The arc of rotation (**Fig. 2**) is suitable for reconstruction of the lower lip, floor of mouth, ventral tongue, and lower one-third of the face.[7] The posteriorly based platysma flap can be used with a supraomohyoid neck dissection or a selective neck dissection that maintains the sternocleidomastoid muscle

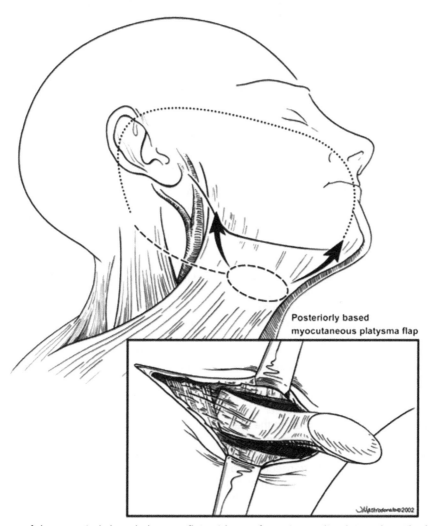

Posteriorly based
myocutaneous platysma flap

Fig. 2. Diagram of the posteriorly based platysma flap with arc of rotation outlined. Note how the fascia associated with the sternocleidomastoid muscle contains the vascular pedicle. (*From* Baur DA. The plastysma myocutaneous flap. Oral Maxillofac Clin North Am 2003;15(4):559–64.)

and its associated fascia, which contains the vascular supply to the platysma.

SURGICAL TECHNIQUE FOR THE POSTERIORLY BASED FLAP

The patient is placed in a supine position with the neck hyperextended and turned to the opposite side. The skin paddle is marked on the ipsilateral submental area, approximating the size of the defect. When designing the flap size, the surgeon must allow for a small amount of primary contracture of the skin paddle.[3] In either version of the platysma flap, the skin paddle can be outlined anywhere within the limits of the muscle. The long axis of the skin paddle should be perpendicular to the muscle fibers. The skin paddle should not cross the midline of the neck to avoid loss of skin at the distal aspect of the flap.[2] Typically, the skin paddle is elliptical in design, but other shapes can be used, depending on the nature of the defect. The long axis of the elliptical skin paddle for an area to cover an intraoral defect should not be smaller than 4 × 3 cm in diameter to ensure inclusion of all of the perforating vessels from the platysma muscle to the skin surface.[7,8] The outlined skin paddle is incised, leaving the platysma muscle intact. A single, horizontal incision extending posteriorly from the already incised skin paddle is made through skin and subcutaneous fat to the level of the platysma muscle, without damaging the muscle. This horizontal incision extends posteriorly past the anterior border of the sternocleidomastoid muscle. Initially, the dissection proceeds cephalad with the elevation of a superior skin flap in the supraplatysmal plane to the inferior border of the mandible. In a similar manner, an inferior skin flap is elevated. One should now be able to visualize almost the entire platysma muscle and the anterior border of the sternocleidomastoid muscle. The skin paddle of the flap should be surrounded by at least 1 cm of platysma muscle circumferentially.[9] After the platysma muscle is fully exposed, mobilization of the myocutaneous flap can be accomplished. The platysma is transected superiorly for its entire anteroposterior length, just below and parallel to the inferior border of the mandible. Care should be taken to avoid the marginal mandibular branch of the facial nerve, which lies in fascia deep to the platysma. In a similar manner, the muscle is horizontally transected inferiorly, parallel to the superior incision, maintaining at least 3 to 4 cm of pedicle width. Anteriorly, any remaining tissue attachment of the muscle is excised. Posteriorly, the flap is now pedicled on the fascia associated with the sternocleidomastoid muscle, in which the vascular supply lies. At

the base of the flap, the external jugular vein should be maintained for venous drainage.[10–14] Once fully mobilized, the flap can be rotated into the defect through a subcutaneous tunnel or into the oral cavity. The donor site is closed in layers after a suction drain is placed. A Burow triangle typically forms at the midline of the neck and often needs to be revised.

SUPERIORLY BASED PLATYSMA FLAP

The dominant blood supply of the superiorly based platysma flap is from the submental branch of the facial artery at or near the inferior border of the mandible, whereas venous drainage is from the submental vein. The submental artery makes numerous anastomoses with the ipsilateral and contralateral lingual, inferior labial, and superior thyroid arteries.[5] Although it is desirable to preserve the facial artery, the flap usually does well even when the ipsilateral facial artery is ligated. The arc of rotation is suitable for reconstruction of the anterior and lateral floor of mouth, buccal mucosa, retromolar trigone, and skin of the lower cheek and parotid region.[7] Motor innervation of the flap may be preserved by maintaining the cervical branch of the facial nerve, assisting with facial animation.[6]

SURGICAL TECHNIQUE

With the neck hyperextended, the proposed skin paddle is outlined on the ipsilateral neck, caudal to the inferior border of the mandible (see **Fig. 2**). The superior incision is made first, and a dissection plane superficial to the platysma muscle is carefully developed cephalad to the inferior border of the mandible. A skin incision is then made at the inferior limb of the skin paddle, with additional exposure of the platysma muscle inferiorly. The platysma muscle is transected sharply at least 1 cm inferior to the edge of the skin paddle, with the subsequent development of a subplatysmal plane of dissection cephalad to just below the inferior border of the mandible. Attention should be paid to the facial arterial perforators, which are located in the proximal part of the flap in the deeper adipofascial plane; the dissection should be deeper at this point to preserve these perforators.

If the cervical branch of the facial nerve is to be incorporated, one must identify the nerve in the superficial layer of the deep cervical fascia and carefully dissect and preserve the proximal portion of the nerve. After both planes of dissection are fully developed, the platysma must be transected vertically, anteriorly, and posteriorly for full mobilization of the flap (**Fig. 3**). As is true for the posteriorly based version, the flap can be introduced into the facial or oral defect by creating an appropriately sized soft tissue tunnel. This tunnel should be of adequate width to avoid strangulating the flap. Care should be taken to avoid twisting the flap or applying excessive traction, which could compromise the vascular supply. The donor site can usually be closed in layers with little difficulty to obtain an acceptable cosmetic result.

DISCUSSION

In any surgical procedure, complications and undesirable sequelae are inevitable. Nevertheless, both versions of the platysma myocutaneous flap are predictable and versatile methods of transferring vascularized tissue to extirpative defects of the oral cavity or lower face. The technique for the development of this flap is straightforward and well within the abilities of most oral and maxillofacial surgeons.

The most dreaded complication of flap surgery is vascular compromise. If the dominant arterial supply is lost, all or a portion of the flap will die. Unlike other axial pattern flaps, such as the pectoralis major flap, the dominant artery is usually not visualized and typically is not mapped with a Doppler study. By carefully staying within the dissection planes and being thoroughly familiar with the anatomy, the surgeon should be able to maintain the integrity of the arterial supply. If, in the postoperative period, the flap appears white with minimal capillary refill, urgently taking the patient back to the operating room will not likely be of benefit, as long as the surgeon is confident that the pedicle was not twisted, strangulated, or excessively stretched.

When the skin paddle appears white in the immediate postoperative period, a skin slough often occurs. Recent studies have reported an incidence of skin slough up to 60%.[15] When this occurs, the underlying muscle usually remains viable. When the flap is used intraorally, the skin

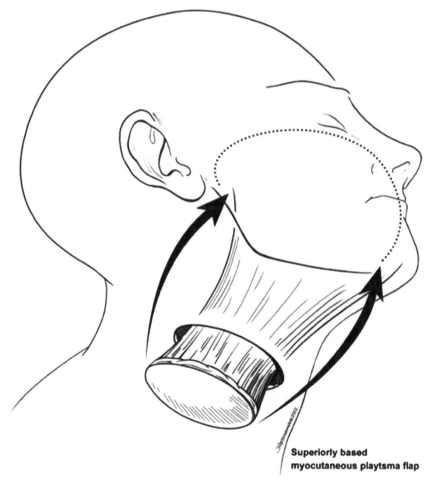

Superiorly based myocutaneous playtsma flap

Fig. 3. Diagram of the superiorly based flap with arc of rotation outlined. (*From* Baur DA. The plastysma myocutaneous flap. Oral Maxillofac Clin North Am 2003;15(4):559–64.)

slough actually allows for mucosalization and a more natural long-term result, with no hair growth in the mouth and the absence of excessive contraction.[3] Skin sloughing can have a more serious esthetic consequence when the flap is used for facial reconstruction. Ariyan[1] reported a case of a platysma muscle flap used for reconstruction of the face, supporting a skin graft after skin slough had occurred. A thorough understanding of the anatomy, especially maintaining an awareness of where the vascular supply enters the pedicle, keeping the vascular pedicle intact, and carefully maintaining the dissection planes without buttonholing the muscle help ensure flap survival. The size of the skin paddle reported in the literature has ranged from 5 × 10 to 7 × 14 cm.[16] Coleman and colleagues[8] recommended designing a large enough skin paddle (at least 5-cm wide) to include several perforators to increase flap survival. Smaller skin paddles may not have enough perforators for adequate skin perfusion[17–19]; however, the authors have used smaller skin paddles with success.

Venous congestion is manifested by a blue, dusky flap. This observation is not an unusual finding, especially in the superiorly based version of the flap, in which venous drainage through the submental vein is poor.[7] In the authors' experience, venous congestion is usually self-limiting, and long-term survival of the flap can be expected. Hematoma formation can be avoided by using a suction drain at the donor site. The drain should be left in place until output drops below 30 mL in a 24-hour period. When the flap is used for oral reconstruction, enteral feeding is performed through a nasogastric tube for 7 to 10 days to protect the flap and to minimize the risk for an oral-cutaneous fistula or a neck infection. The patient is given nothing by mouth until flap closure is ensured. Dehiscence can occur at the recipient site or the donor site. Treatment includes packing the wound and secondary revision as needed. When the platysma flap is raised in conjunction with a neck dissection, there is a theoretical concern for dehiscence at the donor site, because arterial perforators from the platysma to the overlying skin are lost, possibly leading to ischemia at the skin edges and eventual breakdown.[3] If this complication occurs, local wound care or secondary closure result in an acceptable outcome.

Management of the marginal mandibular branch and cervical branch of the facial nerve has already been addressed. Because branches of the cervical nerves are transected during the dissection of either flap, sensation of the neck, postauricular area, or upper chest may be altered; however, these sensory disturbances often diminish with time. The spinal accessory nerve is potentially at risk when the superiorly based version of the platysma flap is used. The spinal accessory nerve is fairly superficial in the posterior triangle of the neck where it enters the anterior border of the trapezius muscle, about 2 to 3 cm superior to the clavicle. Care must be taken when dissecting in this area to avoid damaging the spinal accessory nerve, which could lead to significant shoulder dysfunction, pain, and long-term disability. The reconstructive surgeon has a variety of options for reconstructing defects of the oral cavity and face.[20–22] Functional and esthetic concerns, the size of the defect, donor site morbidity, and the surgeon's level of experience are factors that influence the choice of a reconstructive technique. The posteriorly based and superiorly based versions of the platysma myocutaneous flap have been presented as reliable and versatile techniques of head and neck reconstruction that most oral and maxillofacial surgeons can easily use and incorporate into their reconstructive practice.

SURGICAL PRINCIPLES TO FOLLOW DURING FLAP DEVELOPMENT

By carefully staying within the planes of dissection and being able to preserve the deep adipofascial tissue under the platysma, the surgeon should be able to maintain the integrity of the multiaxial arterial supply.

Avoid excessive torsion, stretching, and suture tension when transposing the flap into the oral cavity. The tunnel for the flap should also be sized properly to prevent strangulation of the flap.

In general, to avoid the risk of compromising blood supply to any random flap, a width to length ratio of 1:3 is the maximum ratio a random flap can tolerate.[23–25]

REFERENCES

1. Ariyan S. The transverse platysma myocutaneous flap for head and neck reconstruction. Plast Reconstr Surg 1997;99(2):340–7.
2. Cannon CR, Johns ME, Atkins JP Jr, et al. Reconstruction of the oral cavity using the platysma myocutaneous flap. Arch Otolaryngol 1982;108(8):491–4.
3. Baur DA, Helman JI. The posteriorly based platysma flap in oral and facial reconstruction: a case series. J Oral Maxillofac Surg 2002;60(10):1147–50.
4. Hollinshead W. The face. In: Harper R, editor. The head and neck anatomy for surgeons. Philadelphia: Lippincott; 1982. p. 293.
5. Hurwitz DJ, Rabson JA, Futrell JW. The anatomic basis for the platysma skin flap. Plast Reconstr Surg 1983;72(3):302–14.

6. Fine NA, Pribaz JJ, Orgill DP. Use of the innervated platysma flap in facial reanimation. Ann Plast Surg 1995;34(3):326–30 [discussion: 330–1].

7. Uehara M, Helman JI, Lillie JH, et al. Blood supply to the platysma muscle flap: an anatomic study with clinical correlation. J Oral Maxillofac Surg 2001; 59(6):642–6.

8. Coleman JJ 3rd, Jurkiewicz MJ, Nahai F, et al. The platysma musculocutaneous flap: experience with 24 cases. Plast Reconstr Surg 1983;72(3):315–23.

9. Banducci DR, Manders EK. Reconstruction of the cheek. In: Baker SR, Swanson NA, editors. Local flaps in facial reconstruction. St Louis (MO): Mosby; 1995. p. 406–9.

10. Cesteleyn L, Helman JI. Facial dissection manual. Ann Arbor, MI: University of Michigan Department of Maxillofacial Surgery; 1998.

11. Li ZN, Li RW, Liu FY, et al. Vertical platysma myocutaneous flap that sacrifices the facial artery and vein. World J Surg Oncol 2013;11(1):165.

12. Wang KH, Hsu EK, Shemen LJ. Platysma myocutaneous flap for oral cavity reconstruction. Ear Nose Throat J 2010;89(6):276–9.

13. Kummoona R. Reconstruction by lateral cervical flap of perioral and oral cavity: clinical and experimental studies. J Craniofac Surg 2010;21(3):660–5.

14. Su T, Zhao YF, Liu B, et al. Clinical review of three types of platysma myocutaneous flap. Int J Oral Maxillofac Surg 2006;35(11):1011–5.

15. Lazaridis N, Dimitrakopoulos I, Zouloumis L. The superiorly based platysma flap for oral reconstruction in conjunction with neck dissection: a case series. J Oral Maxillofac Surg 2007;65(5):895–900.

16. Futrell JW, Johns ME, Edgerton MT, et al. Platysma myocutaneous flap for intraoral reconstruction. Am J Surg 1978;136(4):504–7.

17. Howaldt HP, Bitter K. The myocutaneous platysma flap for the reconstruction of intraoral defects after radical tumour resection. J Craniomaxillofac Surg 1989;17(5):237–40.

18. Szudek J, Taylor SM. Systematic review of the platysma myocutaneous flap for head and neck reconstruction. Arch Otolaryngol Head Neck Surg 2007; 133(7):655–61.

19. Tosco P, Garzino-Demo P, Ramieri G, et al. The platysma myocutaneous flap (PMF) for head and neck reconstruction: a retrospective and multicentric analysis of 91 T1-T2 patients. J Craniomaxillofac Surg 2012;40(8):e415–8.

20. Papadopoulos ON, Gamatsi IE. Platysma myocutaneous flap for intraoral and surface reconstruction. Ann Plast Surg 1993;31(1):15–8.

21. Edgerton MT, Desprez JD. Reconstruction of the oral cavity in the treatment of cancer. Plast Reconstr Surg (1946) 1957;19(2):89–113.

22. Desprez JD, Kiehn CL. Methods of reconstruction following resection of anterior oral cavity and mandible for malignancy. Plast Reconstr Surg Transplant Bull 1959;24:238–49.

23. Shah AR, Rosenberg D. Defining the facial extent of the platysma muscle: a review of 71 consecutive face-lifts. Arch Facial Plast Surg 2009;11(6): 405–8.

24. Cartier C, Jouzdani E, Garrel R, et al. Study of the platysma coli muscle vascularisation by the facial artery. Implication during the elevation of the musculocutaneous platysma coli muscle flap. Rev Laryngol Otol Rhinol (Bord) 2009;130(3):139–44 [in French].

25. Imanishi N, Nakajima H, Kishi K, et al. Is the platysma flap musculocutaneous? Angiographic study of the platysma. Plast Reconstr Surg 2005;115(4): 1018–24.

The Use of Cervicofacial Flap in Maxillofacial Reconstruction

 CrossMark

Anastasios Sakellariou, DMD, MD*,
Andrew Salama, DDS, MD

KEYWORDS

- Cervicofacial flap • Maxillofacial surgery • Cheek defects • Temporofrontal defects • Brow defects
- Platysma muscle

KEY POINTS

- The cervicofacial (CF) flap offers an excellent texture and color match with the recipient area.
- This flap can be used for defects of the cheek, temple, and orbit.
- The surgeon may extend the plane of dissection deep to the superficial musculoaponeurotic system (SMAS) and platysma muscle in order to improve the blood supply of the transferred tissue.
- The flap can be used alone or in combination with regional and free flaps depending on the extent of the defect.

INTRODUCTION

The human cheek occupies most of the middle third of the face and is an important subunit for oromandibular function and form, while the need for reconstruction often stems from neoplastic or traumatic causes. The midface, because of its prominent position, is susceptible to ultraviolet radiation and traumatic injury, and reconstructing a defect in this region can pose a challenge to any maxillofacial surgeon. Although full-thickness defects often require free flap reconstruction, a partial-thickness defect can be repaired with a myriad of local and regional flap techniques.

The decision in selecting an appropriate flap for cheek reconstruction can be a daunting task. Roth and colleagues[1] divided the cheek into 3 zones to help determine the method of cheek reconstruction (**Fig. 1**). Zones II and III provide the most opportunities for direct closure, especially in elderly patients. Zone I, however, carries a unique challenge because of the proximity of the nearby vital structures. Inappropriate flap selection in Zone I reconstruction can lead to significant esthetic and functional deformities (ie, ectropion). One of the most reliable flaps in reconstructing defects in this region is the CF flap.

The first published local flap method reported for cheek reconstruction was in 1918 by Esser.[2] Since then, various methods have been described in the literature, many of which have the disadvantage of creating prominent scars. One of the most useful reconstructive techniques in repairing cheek defect is the CF flap.[3–5] The CF flap in its modern form was first described by Juri and Juri.[6] Conceptually, it is a random, rotation-advancement flap that exploits the skin laxity of the cheek, preauricular region, and neck. The main advantage of the flap is that the color and texture match those of the native tissue (**Box 1**). Another major advantage is that the surgical incisions can be more inconspicuous and follow the borders of the facial subunits. The flap also allows adequate exposure of the CF structures for

Oral and Maxillofacial Surgery Department, Boston University, 100 East Newton Street, Boston, MA 02118, USA
* Corresponding author.
E-mail address: Anastasios.Sakellariou@bmc.org

Oral Maxillofacial Surg Clin N Am 26 (2014) 389–400
http://dx.doi.org/10.1016/j.coms.2014.05.007
1042-3699/14/$ – see front matter © 2014 Elsevier Inc. All rights reserved.

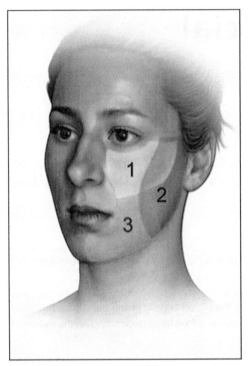

Fig. 1. The 3 unique zones considered in cheek reconstruction. (*Adapted from* Roth DA, Longaker MT, Zide BM. Cheek surface reconstruction: best choices according to zones. Operat Tech Plast Reconstr Surg 1998;5(1):26–36.)

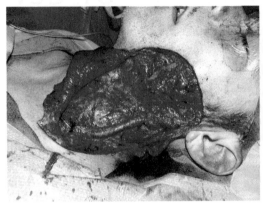

Fig. 2. Neck exposure allowing lymph node dissection.

additional oncologic procedures, such as lymph node dissection and parotidectomy (**Fig. 2**).

INDICATIONS

The defect size, depth, and location are the main factors dictating the treatment plan (**Box 2**). The CF flap is ideal for large defects that cannot be addressed with small, local tissue mobilization but are not extensive enough to require free tissue transfer. Superomedial cheek defects (Zone I) larger than 3 to 4 cm typically fall into this category. The

use of the CF flap is commonly confined to the cutaneous layer of reconstruction. In addition to midface reconstruction, the CF flap has been used alone or in combination with other techniques to restore defects in the upper third of the face,[7–9] defects after orbital exenteration,[10,11] and through-and-through cheek defects.[12–15]

CONTRAINDICATIONS

Active skin infections should delay the use of this reconstructive modality. The CF flap must be performed on healthy tissue in order to decrease the risk of complications and optimize esthetic results.

Severe systemic comorbidities that increase the perioperative risk are also contraindications. However, the CF flap can be performed under local anesthesia. Lidocaine (1%) with 1:100,000 epinephrine can provide profound analgesia to patients whose physical status precludes general anesthesia. Although a history of smoking is known to increase wound complication rates in dermatologic and facial skin flap surgery,[16] it alone is not a contraindication to the use of the CF flap. Caution should be exercised in flap design in this patient population. Previous radiation to the surgical site should also be considered as a relative contraindication.[13]

Box 1
Advantages

- Excellent color and texture match.
- Camouflage scars in the cheek borders.
- The ability to be performed under local anesthesia.
- Ease of harvesting.
- Proximity to the defect.
- Minimal morbidity.

Box 2
Indications

- Partial-thickness cheek defects (usually 3 to 4 cm and up to 10 cm).
- Temporofrontal and brow defects.[10,11]
- Orbital exenteration defects.[12–15]

ANATOMY
The Cheek

The cheek is a laminated structure composed of superficial to deep layers: epidermis, dermis, subcutaneous tissue, and the SMAS. Deeper structures include branches of the facial nerve, the parotid gland, the buccal fat pad, and the mandible, inferiorly. The facial nerve branches are protected beneath the SMAS in most locations. Thus, a surgeon who prefers dissection beneath the SMAS layer must be familiar with the facial nerve anatomy.

The borders of the cheek with the other subunits are essential in camouflaging the scar lines, including the infraorbital rim, nasolabial fold, preauricular crease, and inferior mandibular margin.

SMAS

Understanding the anatomy of the SMAS is of utmost importance for the facial surgeon. The SMAS was first described by Mitz and Peyronie[17] in 1976, and the extended craniofacial tissue encloses the platysma, risorius, triangularis, auricularis, occipitalis, and frontalis muscles. SMAS is connected to the dermis by fibrous septae allowing movement of the skin during facial expressions. The SMAS is confluent with the galea layer on the scalp and with the temporoparietal fascia in the temporal region. In the neck, the SMAS continues as the superficial cervical fascia. The surgical importance of the SMAS lies in its relationship with the facial nerve. The motor nerves are found deep to the fascia, whereas the sensory branches are located superficial to it.

The vascularity of the SMAS has been of debate for many years. Although anatomic studies report that the SMAS is an avascular layer, there is clinical evidence suggesting otherwise. Schaverien and colleagues[18] used sequential dying and 3-dimensional computed tomographic angiography and venography on 24 hemifaces. The investigators found that the SMAS is perfused by the transverse facial artery perforator branches on their route to the subdermal plexus. This finding is supported by the observation that skin necrosis is more frequently encountered in subcutaneous face-lifts where the SMAS is not included in the flap.

Flap Anatomy

Arterial supply
The blood supplies for the CF flap can be divided into 2 portions: (1) facial and (2) neck portions. The facial portion of the flap is dissected in the subcutaneous level, which receives its blood supply via the subdermal plexus in a random pattern.

A modification of this portion of the flap to incorporate the SMAS has been proposed by Kroll and colleagues[19] to enhance the vascularity by providing the flap with an axial blood supply (via perforators from the transverse facial artery). The neck portion of the flap, on the other hand, is dissected in a subplatysmal plane. By doing so, the platysma serves as a blood supply to this region. The platysma (**Box 3**), as described by Hurwitz and colleagues,[20] is a muscle supplied by the occipital and postauricular arteries posteriorly, the submental artery superiorly and medially, the superior thyroid artery centrally, and the CF trunk inferiorly. However, during flap elevation, only the perforators from the submental artery are preserved.

Venous drainage
The flap's venous drainage is provided by the external jugular vein and randomized dermal venous drainage. Enclosing the external jugular vein in the flap helps to decrease the risk of venous congestion and ischemic necrosis.

Innervation
Sensory innervation is provided by branches of the greater auricular (C2–C3) and lesser occipital (C2) nerves. Careful dissection reduces the risk of paresthesia, and patients should be informed of this potential complication.

The facial nerve exists in the stylomastoid foramen and travels within the parenchyma of the parotid gland to reach the muscles of facial expression. The facial nerve is further divided into 5 major branches. Among the 5 branches, the temporal and marginal mandibular branches are more susceptible to iatrogenic surgery because of the lack of collateral innervation. The nerve can be found beneath the SMAS in the face and platysma in the neck, and the approximate course of the temporal branch can be traced by following the Pitanguy line (from a point 0.5 cm below the tragus to a point 1.5 cm lateral to the supraorbital rim).[21]

Box 3
Arterial supply to the platysma

- Occipital
- Postauricular
- Submental
- Superior thyroid
- Cervicofacial trunk

Data from Hurwitz DJ, Rabson JA, Futrell JW. The anatomic basis for the platysma skin flap. Plast Reconstr Surg 1983;72:302–12.

The marginal mandibular nerve anterior to the facial artery travels exclusively above the inferior border of the mandible. Posterior to the artery, it is found below the mandible in 19% of the cases (**Fig. 3**).[22]

PREOPERATIVE PLANNING
Patient Evaluation

Local
Preoperative planning includes local and systemic evaluations. Qualities such as skin laxity, color, tone, and texture warrant consideration because they may greatly affect the esthetic outcome. Patients with decreased skin laxity, sebaceous skin, higher grading in the Fitzpatrick classification, or a history of keloids may present a greater operative challenge. Therefore, a detailed conversation with the patient regarding realistic expectations is essential.

Local factors, such as the size, depth, and relation of the defect to the adjacent structures largely influence surgical planning. Full-thickness defects, for example, require the addition of a free or a regional flap such as the temporal muscle flap, in order to meet ideal reconstructive goals. Defects of considerable size require extending the flap margins to the pectoral region to minimize skin tension and to decrease the risk of dehiscence.

Systemic
The systemic effects of tobacco smoking are an important consideration in local and regional flaps; smoking impedes cutaneous wound healing via various mechanisms.[12] Vasoconstriction by 30% to 40%, thrombosis in the microvasculature, as well as endothelial and fibroblast dysfunction are only a few of the wide spectrum of physiologic changes associated with tobacco smoking. These effects can clinically translate into skin necrosis, infection, and dehiscence. Although there is no consensus regarding the recommended duration of cessation, cessation of smoking 2 weeks preoperatively and 1 week postoperatively may reduce complication rates.

A standard preoperative physical status classification according to the American Society of Anesthesiologists is indicated in individuals of older age and those with comorbidities. As mentioned above, local anesthesia can be used for patients who are poor candidates for general anesthesia. Local anesthetic infiltration offers good analgesia, hemostasis, and a plane of hydrodissection that helps facilitate flap elevation.

PROCEDURE
Preparation and Positioning

Antibiotic prophylaxis may be used, depending on the cause of the defect. A single, weight-based, intravenous dose of first-generation cephalosporin for skin bacteria coverage is a reasonable choice, and clindamycin is an alternative antibiotic in the case of allergic reaction history. A standard sterile skin preparation for maxillofacial procedures is applied and should include the bilateral neck and chest. A gel-padded head stabilizer and shoulder roll help with exposure and positioning; the latter provides the necessary skin tension and facilitates the incision and dissection of the flap via neck extension. However, a history of severe cervical rheumatoid arthritis or cervical spine trauma should first be excluded.

Technique

Incision and design
Multiple variations and modifications of the CF flap have been described since it was initially introduced. The classic design, as described by Juri and Juri,[6] is an advancement-rotational, inferomedially based flap. The incision design of this flap is similar to that used in CF rhytidectomy, in which the incision is marked and 1% lidocaine with 1:100,000 epinephrine is injected into the subcutaneous plane. The incision starts with a #15 blade at the most inferior part of the nasolabial groove and travels upward lateral to the defect. Then, from the lateral canthus, the incision is extended outward along the zygomatic arch to the hairline and preauricular crease. Finally, it loops around the earlobe and continues along the hairline (**Fig. 4**). Depending on the location of the defect, the flap may have different cephalad and caudad extensions (**Fig. 5**). A pectoral extension[13,14] is

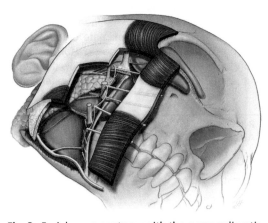

Fig. 3. Facial nerve anatomy with the surrounding tissues in 3-dimensions. (*From* Mendelson BC, Wong CH. Anatomy of the aging face. In: Warren RJ, Neligan PC, editors. Plastic surgery. 3rd edition. vol. 2. Edinburgh (United Kingdom): Saunders; 2012. p. 85; with permission.)

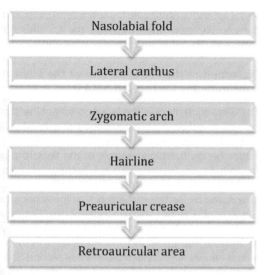

Fig. 4. Sequence of incision for laterally based cervico-facial flap.

often needed to improve flap mobility (**Fig. 6**). It is important to mention, here, that the cheek's RSTLs change from horizontal to vertical orientation as one moves from the medial to the lateral areas.

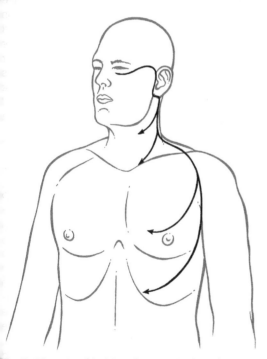

Fig. 5. Diagram of incisions for anterior-based cervico-facial and cervicopectoral flaps, with back-cuts oriented in a cervical crease, in the supraclavicular region, above the areola, and along the costal margin. (*From* Mureau MA, Hofer SO. Maximizing results in reconstruction of cheek defects. Clin Plast Surg 2009;36:461–76; with permission.)

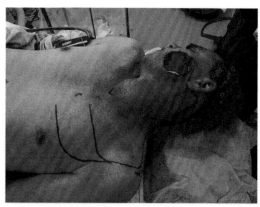

Fig. 6. Clinical picture showing different inferior extensions of the flap.

Dissection

Cephalad to the zygomatic arch, the dissection is kept in the subcutaneous plane to avoid injury to the frontal branches of the facial nerve. In the parotid region, the dissection can remain in the subcutaneous layer, as found in the conventional CF flap, or incorporate the SMAS in the deep-plane cervicofacial flap. Care should be taken to avoid nerve injury in the area anterior to the parotid gland, where the facial nerve branches are no longer protected by the gland. The use of a fine hemostat or McCabe dissector for blunt dissection and bipolar diathermy reduces the risk of nerve damage.

As the dissection approaches the inferior border of the mandible, one should be aware of the location of the marginal mandibular branch of the facial nerve. In this case, a nerve stimulator can be used to localize the facial nerve. When elevating the neck portion of the flap, the authors advocate the inclusion of the platysma muscle for better blood supply. The importance of including platysma in this portion of the flap has been demonstrated in Hakim and colleagues' study.[23] Thus, the flap components vary by anatomic location:

- Superior to the zygomatic arch: flap contains skin and subcutaneous tissue.
- Inferior to the zygomatic arch: flap contains skin, subcutaneous tissue, and the SMAS.
- The cervical portion is composed of the platysma and skin layers.

Therefore, the SMAS dissection must be converted to the subplatysmal plane at the inferior border of the mandible.

The dissection is continued anteriorly and inferiorly until adequate mobilization and tension-free closure of the defect are achieved upon advancing and rotating the flap (**Fig. 7**). The skin

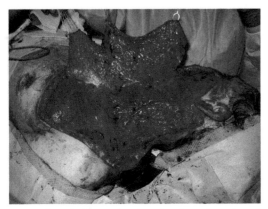

Fig. 7. Clinical picture showing the dissection of cervicothoracic flap and its mobility.

defect is now transferred to the neck where primary closure usually suffices by exploiting the skin's laxity.

Closure

The wound should be closed in a tension-free manner. The authors use 3-0 Vicryl suture (Ethicon Inc, Somerville, NJ, USA) for subcutaneous tissue and 5-0 Monocryl suture (Ethicon Inc) for the skin in a subcuticular manner. Steri-Strips (3M, Maplewood, MN, USA) are placed after the application of a compound of benzoin tincture. In the neck and thorax, staples are used, and drains are placed only if necessary. A closed drain to suction (Jackson-Pratt) is the authors' preference, because it has a lower risk of contamination.

MODIFICATIONS
Increased Arc of Rotation

The modern CF flap consists of facial and cervical portions; however, when a greater arc of rotation is needed, a pectoral extension can be used. The cervicothoracic (CT) flap was first described by Conley[3] in 1960, and later coined by Garrett and colleagues[5] in 1966. In addition to the blood supplies for the CF flap, the CT flap also includes blood supply via perforators from the internal mammary artery. The facial and cervical portions of the flap are raised in a similar manner to those found in the conventional CF flap, and the pectoral portion of the flap is raised in the subcutaneous layer. An inferior extension of the CT flap can extend to the level of the costal margin, but most studies recommend its termination at a level above the areola. The medial extent of the flap in the chest should be 2 cm lateral to the sternal border, in order to preserve the internal mammary perforators. While comparing the CT flap with the conventional CF flap, Moore and colleagues[13]

and Liu and colleagues[14] separately compared the complication rates between the CF and CT flaps and did not appreciate any difference.

Dissection in the Facial Portion of the Flap: Subcutaneous Versus Sub-SMAS

The dissection plane in the facial portion of the flap can be in either the subcutaneous or sub-SMAS levels. The incorporation of the SMAS can theoretically change the blood supply of the flap from a random to an axial pattern via perforators from the transverse facial artery. This benefit was first advocated by Barton and Zilmer[24] at the American Society of Plastic and Reconstructive Surgery meeting in 1982 (**Table 1**) and later published by Kroll and colleagues[19] in 1994. However, this theoretical benefit was challenged in Whetzel and Stevenson's[25] cadaver study. In this study, the investigators found no difference in the blood supply based on ink-injection patterns between the skin flaps that were elevated with or without SMAS incorporation. Clinically, Jacono and colleagues[26] conducted a retrospective study to compare these 2 techniques in relation to their complication rates. The study found no difference in skin necrosis, except in patients who have history of tobacco smoking. Moreover, dissection beneath the SMAS layer likely increases the risk of injuring the facial nerve. The intimacy of the nerve to the SMAS and the relatively high success rate of the subcutaneous version of this flap in the literature have many surgeons questioning the legitimacy of SMAS incorporation.

Reverse CF Flap

The design, as described above, refers to the forward CF advancement-rotation flap. Alternatively, the reverse CF flap can be used. In this schema, the pedicle is located in the preauricular area, and the arc of rotation is superolateral. The incision starts at the medial aspect of the defect, descending along the melolabial sulcus, and extending to the

Table 1		
Advantages and disadvantages of deep-plane cervicofacial flap		
Advantages	**Disadvantages**	
Better vascularization	Facial nerve injury	
Better mobility	More operating time	
Thicker	More technically	
More adaptable	challenging	

Adapted from Delay E, Lucas R, Jorquera F. Composite cervicofacial flap for reconstruction of complex cheek defects. Ann Plast Surg 1999;43:347–53.

neck following the facial subunit boundaries to ensure scar camouflage (**Fig. 8**). The flap is elevated and superiorly advanced to close the defect.

Boyette and Vural[27] advocate the use of the reverse flap for superomedial cheek defects in which the horizontal axis is greater than the vertical one (**Fig. 9**). The investigators described its use in 6 cases with a mean flap size of 6 × 4.9 cm and reported no flap failures. Three of the patients had postoperative ectropion without necessitating surgical treatment. The investigators opine that a reverse CF flap for horizontally oriented defects helps to decrease flap tension and minimize excessive skin excision for standing cone deformities.

Technique for Temporofrontal Defects

A CF flap has been described to reconstruct large temporoparietal and brow defects.[7–9] In this case, the local advancement flap is limited because of the unfavorable migration of hair-bearing structures into normally glabrous skin, whereas in the scalp or free flap transfer, the donor tissue is usually too thick, which can lead to eyelid distortion. The CF flap is devoid of the above disadvantages and offers an excellent color and texture match. Cole and colleagues[8] reported 3 cases of using CF flaps in repairing this region, and all cases had satisfactory results.

For the reconstruction of temporofrontal defects, the incision begins at the cephalolateral area of the defect. The incision is then directed laterally along the hairline until it reaches the preauricular crease. At this point, the incision is carried caudally to the neck; it is important to follow a relaxed skin tension line in the neck.

Superior to the zygomatic arch, the dissection is kept in the subcutaneous plane. Inferior to the zygomatic arch, the dissection follows a deeper plane, including the SMAS, to enhance the flap's blood supply. The use of blunt dissection and bipolar electrocautery are essential to minimize tissue trauma and nerve injuries. After adequate elevation and mobilization, the flap is rotated and advanced to close the temporofrontal and brow defects. If the defect size is significant, a second flap should be used.

Alternatively, D'Arpa and colleagues[9] described a method for the reconstruction of temporal defects. The investigators overlap (plication) the SMAS layer to allow a further cranial advancement of the CF flap. After performing a face-lift type of incision, dissection over the SMAS is used with face-lift scissors. After flap elevation, purse-string sutures are placed to tighten the SMAS and bring it superiorly. With this maneuver, tension-free closure can be achieved easily and tissue advancement is maximized. These purse-string sutures are not anchored to the deeper

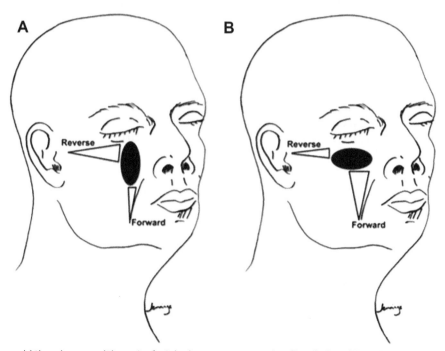

Fig. 8. Forward (*A*) and reverse (*B*) cervicofacial advancement-rotation flap design. (*From* Boyette JR, Vural E. Cervicofacial advancement-rotation flap in midface reconstruction: forward or reverse? Otolaryngol Head Neck Surg 2011;144:196–200; with permission.)

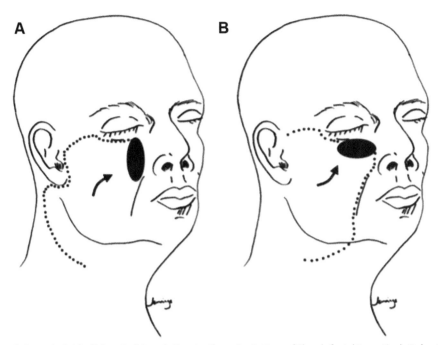

Fig. 9. Size of discarded skin (triangles) in relation to the orientation of the defect (*A*, vertical; *B*, horizontal) for forward and reverse flaps. (*Data from* Boyette JR, Vural E. Cervicofacial advancement-rotation flap in midface reconstruction: forward or reverse? Otolaryngol Head Neck Surg 2011;144:196–200; with permission.)

tissue, which helps the tissue to migrate inferiorly as healing progresses and assists in alleviating any asymmetry that has been created. After the passing of the purse-string sutures, any irregularities are corrected by tissue defatting.

Orbital Exenteration

Orbital exenteration is indicated when malignancy has violated the orbital contents.[10,11] The reconstructive goals for these patients are (1) to separate paranasal sinus and intracranial contents from the orbital defect and (2) to provide cutaneous lining that can tolerate radiation therapy and accommodate prosthetic rehabilitation.[28] Skin grafts, regional flaps from the temporal arterial system, and free flaps are common reconstructive modalities for orbital exenteration. Many of these modalities carry their own advantages and disadvantages. Alternatively, the CF flap has been proposed as a treatment option. With its ease of harvesting, proximity to the defect, and similar skin color and texture to the surrounding tissue, the CF flap is a good option. Rabey and colleagues[10] and Cuesta-Gil and colleagues[11] both reported acceptable results using CF flaps for this indication.

POSTOPERATIVE CARE

Patients should rest with the head elevated for the first few days after surgery. The dressings should be removed on the second postoperative day because, by that time, the wound healing would have sealed the dead space from the overlying skin surface. Drains are removed when their output is less than 20 mL in a 24 hour period. It is important that the patient keeps the incisions clean and free of dried blood with a sterile barrier. There is no indication for postoperative antibiotic coverage. It is of utmost importance that the sutures are removed within 5 days to avoid railroad track marking on the skin if a subcuticular technique is not used.

COMPLICATIONS

Proper patient selection, gentle tissue handling, and adequate hemostasis minimize the complication rate. General surgical complications, such as hematoma formation and infection, are treated with evacuation, drainage, and antibiotic coverage. Hematomas require immediate attention because they jeopardize the blood supply of the flap, potentiating the risk of necrosis. Specific complications related to the CF flap are standing cone deformity, long-term ectropion, distal tip necrosis (DTN), and nerve injuries (**Table 2**).

Standing cone deformity or dog-ear refers to the excess tissue occurring at the end of the closure after skin transposition; it is a cosmetic problem that is better addressed with surgical excision at the time of the surgery.

Table 2
Complication rate

Study, Year	Number of Patients	Age	Average Size	Flap Type	Risk Factor	Distal End Necrosis	Ectropion	Facial Nerve Paralysis
Cook et al,[37] 1991	14	51	3.9 × 4.3 cm	SC-CF	Smoker: 35% Radiation: 29%	2 (14%)	1 (7%)	0
Becker et al,[33] 1996	5 (35 flaps)	NA	NA	Sub-SMAS CF	NA	1 (20%)	2 (40%)	0
Tan et al,[34] 2005	18	76.7	5.6 × 5.3 cm	Sub-SMAS CF	Smoker: 5% Radiation: 17%	1 (5%)	2 (11%)	0
Moore et al,[13] 2005	33	65.9	NA	SC-CF: 20 SC-CT: 15	Smoker: 77% Radiation: 71%	8 (23%) superficial 3 (10%) full thickness	3 (8.5%)	0
Austen et al,[36] 2009	32	71	7.2 × 5.8 cm	SC-CF	Smoker: 16% Radiation: 9%	3 (9%)	1 (3%)	0
Boyette & Vural,[27] 2011	13	59.8	4.9 × 4.5 cm	SC-CF	Smoker: 62%	0 (0%)	6 (46%)	0
Liu et al,[14] 2011	21	64.5	6.5 × 3.9 cm	SC-CF: 10 SC-CT: 11	NA	3 (14.3%): superficial 2 (9.5%): full thickness	NA	NA
Rapstine et al,[30] 2012	82	60	NA	SC-CF	Smoker: 25%	2 (2.4%)	5 (6%)	NA
Jacono et al,[26] 2014	88	65	SC-CF: 12.9 cm² Sub-SMAS: 18.8 cm²	SC-CF: 69 (78%) Sub-SMAS: 19 (22%)	Smoker: 18 (20%)	24 (27%) • All in SC group	3 (3%) • All in SC group	0
Ebrahimi & Nejadsarvari,[38] 2013	30	52.9	2.76 × 8.0 cm	SC-CF	NA	0	0	NA
Total	336 (338 flaps)	63.1	23.24 cm²	SC-CF: 296 flaps Sub-SMAS-CF: 42 flaps	—	49 (14.5%) • SC: 47/296 (15%) • Sub-SMAS: 2/42 (4.7%)	23 (6.8%)	0%

Abbreviations: SC-CF, subcutaneous CF; SC-CT, subcutaneous CT.

Postoperative ectropion occurs when the flap is extended to the infraorbital region. Postoperative edema forces the eversion of the lower eyelid, and as healing proceeds, scarring and fibrosis may maintain the eyelid in this everted position. The incidence rate of ectropion is approximately 6.8%. Extending the flap superiorly to the lateral canthus and suturing it to the periosteum reduce the risk of persistent ectropion. Another way to prevent this complication is the use of frost suture.[29] A nylon 4-0 suture is passed through the tarsal plate and then secured at the supraorbital region. The free ends are then joined and form a sling counteracting the caudal tension. An additional way to prevent ectropion is the use of the Yin-Yang rotation, as described by Belmahi and colleagues,[7] for cases in which minimal skin laxity is appreciated. In this technique, a temporoparietal scalp flap is raised and rotated in the opposite direction of the CF flap to close the preauricular cutaneous defect. Raising the additional temporoparietal scalp flap helps to minimize wound tension and provide cephalic anchorage to the facial flap, which decreases the incidence of ectropion.

DTN may occur due to the unreliable random pattern of the flap vascularization (**Fig. 10**). DTN may also contribute to the decreased blood supply associated with thinner skin in the older oncologic population. The incidence rate from the published literature is approximately 14.5%, and risk factors associated with DTN include a history of smoking, radiation therapy, and diabetes. Although raising the flap with the SMAS can theoretically increase the blood supply, clinical study has not yet found its validity. Incorporating the SMAS for patients without risk factors may not provide additional benefits, but those with associated risk factors may find significant improvement as demonstrated in the study by Jacono and colleagues.[26] Another measure to avoid DTN is to include the external jugular vein with the flap to improve the

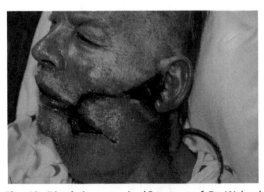

Fig. 10. Distal tip necrosis. (*Courtesy of* Dr Waleed Ezzat, Boston, MA, USA.)

venous outflow of the flap. Moreover, when the flap tension is unavoidable because of the size of the defect, additional grafts or flaps are necessary.

Facial nerve injury is a dreadful complication that leads to major functional and esthetic deficits. In-depth knowledge of the facial anatomy, blunt dissection, and the use of bipolar electrocautery are the mainstays of prevention, as discussed in the surgical technique section. Published studies have found relatively low incidence rates of facial injury, and when it occurs, it is usually transient. Facial nerve injury should be first managed with conservative therapy (oral steroid and close follow-up). Persistent paralysis after 6 months without improvement may warrant facial reanimation surgery.

DISCUSSION

The CF flap is a well-tested technique for reconstructing moderate to large upper and midfacial defects. In a case series of 400 cheek reconstruction,[30] the CF flap was the second most common flap to be used. Most of these defects are located in Zone 1 and are partial-thickness defects, and the size of the defect is greater than 2 cm. The popularity of this flap mostly stems from its advantages in the ease of harvesting, minimal postoperative morbidity, versatility in flap design, great arc of rotation, and similar color and texture with the surrounding tissue.

Versatility in flap design and a great arc of rotation allow CF flaps to cover large areas of defect. The conventional CF flap is laterally based and used mostly to cover medial cheek defects. Since its initial report, multiple modifications have been published. Haddock and Zide[31] as well as Longaker and colleagues[32] have reported the use of the CF flap as a medially based flap to reconstruct large lateral cheek defects. In addition, the inferior extension of the flap below the clavicle was advocated to increase the arc of rotation. All these contributions have helped the CF flap remain a viable option for any reconstructive surgeon.

Like any surgical technique, controversy does exist in terms of the most appropriate plane of dissection in the facial portion of the flap. However, no study has shown a superiority of one technique over the other. Perhaps the decision on which technique to use should be based on the patient's risk factors and surgeon's experience. As noted in Jacono and colleagues'[26] study, patients with smoking or irradiated histories benefit from sub-SMAS dissection, whereas low-risk patients may do just fine with the subcutaneous CF flap. The second factor is associated with the surgeon's experience. Owing to the intimacy of this flap with the facial nerve, those unfamiliar with facial anatomy should raise it subcutaneously to prevent iatrogenic injury to the nerve. Although studies[25,33,34] did not find higher incidence rates of facial injury with sub-SMAS dissection, one should be cautious in interpreting the results of these studies. Surgeries performed in these studies are usually conducted by experienced surgeons, which may lead to a more favorable outcome. In the era of highly successful free flap reconstruction, experiences with CF flaps are difficult to accumulate; however, those who have performed composite rhytidectomy as described by Hamra[35] find dissection of the sub-SMAS CF flap to be similar.

The indications of CF flaps are most often applied in a partial-thickness defect. Reports of its use, together with other flaps for full-thickness defects, have been published. Both temporalis[12] and pectoralis flaps[13,14] have been used together with CF flaps to reconstruct through-and-through cheek defects. This reconstructive option is particularly important for patients who have depleted neck vessels for free flap reconstruction. Moreover, the CF flap can also be used together with a free flap for complex reconstruction. This combination eliminates the need for double free flaps in these cases. Bianchi and colleagues[15] report the use of the CF flap in combination with an iliac crest flap for the treatment of a T4N0M0 lip squamous cell carcinoma (SCC) and with a fibular osseocutaneous free flap for the treatment of a T4N0M0 oral floor SCC. Both cases provide good results. Although by no means can a CF flap replace free flap reconstruction when needed, it can serve as a good treatment alternative.

REFERENCES

1. Roth DA, Longaker MT, Zide BM. Cheek surface reconstruction: best choices according to zones. Operat Tech Plast Reconstr Surg 1998;5(1):26–36.
2. Esser JF. Rotation der Wange. Leipzig (Germany): Vogel; 1918.
3. Conley J. The use of regional flaps in head and neck surgery. Ann Otol Rhinol Laryngol 1960;69:1223–34.
4. Mustarde JC. Repair and reconstruction in the orbital region. 2nd edition. London: Churchill-Livingstone; 1980.
5. Garrett WS, Giblin TR, Hoffman GW. Closure of skin defects of the face and neck by rotation and advancement of cervicopectoral flaps. Plast Reconstr Surg 1966;38(4):342–6.
6. Juri J, Juri C. Advancement and rotation of a large cervicofacial flap for cheek repairs. Plast Reconstr Surg 1979;64(5):692–6.
7. Belmahi A, Oufkir A, Bron T, et al. Reconstruction of cheek skin defects by the 'Yin-Yang' rotation of the Mustardé flap and the temporoparietal scalp. J Plast Reconstr Aesthet Surg 2009;62(4):506–9.
8. Cole EL, Sanchez ER, Ortiz DA, et al. Expanded indications for the deep plane cervicofacial flap: aesthetic reconstruction of large combined temporofrontal and brow defects. Ann Plast Surg 2013. [E-pub ahead of print].
9. D'Arpa S, Cordova A, Pirrello R, et al. The face lift SMAS plication flap for reconstruction of large temporofrontal defects: reconstructive surgery meets cosmetic surgery. Plast Reconstr Surg 2011; 127(5):2068–75.
10. Rabey N, Abood A, Gillespie P, et al. Reconstruction of complex orbital exenteration defects. Ann Plast Surg 2013. [E-pub ahead of print].
11. Cuesta-Gil M, Concejo C, Acero J, et al. Repair of large orbito-cutaneous defects by combining two classical flaps. J Craniomaxillofac Surg 2004;32(1):21–7.
12. Helman JI. The cervicofacial flap in facial reconstruction. Oral Maxillofac Surg Clin North Am 2003; 15(4):551–7.
13. Moore BA, Wine T, Netterville JL. Cervicofacial and cervicothoracic rotation flaps in head and neck reconstruction. Head Neck 2005;27(12):1092–101.
14. Liu FY, Xu ZF, Li P, et al. The versatile application of cervicofacial and cervicothoracic rotation flaps in head and neck surgery. World J Surg Oncol 2011; 9(1):135.
15. Bianchi B, Ferri A, Ferrari S, et al. Free and locoregional flap associations in the reconstruction of extensive head and neck defects. Int J Oral Maxillofac Surg 2008;37(8):723–9.
16. Calhoun KH, Kinsella JB, Hokanson JA, et al. Smoking increases facial skin flap complications. Otolaryngol Head Neck Surg 1995;113(2):P56.
17. Mitz V, Peyronie M. The superficial musculoaponeurotic system (SMAS) in the parotid and cheek area. Plast Reconstr Surg 1976;58(1):80–8.
18. Schaverien MV, Pessa JE, Saint-Cyr M, et al. The arterial and venous anatomies of the lateral face lift flap and the SMAS. Plast Reconstr Surg 2009; 123(5):1581–7.
19. Kroll SS, Reece GP, Robb G, et al. Deep-plane cervicofacial rotation-advancement flap for reconstruction of large cheek defects. Plast Reconstr Surg 1994;94(1):88–93.
20. Hurwitz DJ, Rabson JA, Futrell JW. The anatomic basis for the platysma skin flap. Plast Reconstr Surg 1983;72(3):302–12.
21. Pitanguy I, Ramos AS. The frontal branch of the facial nerve. Plast Reconstr Surg 1966;38(4):352–6.
22. Dingman RO, Grabb WC. Surgical anatomy of the mandibular ramus of the facial nerve based on the

dissection of 100 facial halves. Plast Reconstr Surg 1962;29(3):266–72.

23. Hakim SG, Jacobsen HC, Aschoff HH, et al. Including the platysma muscle in a cervicofacial skin rotation flap to enhance blood supply for reconstruction of vast orbital and cheek defects: anatomical considerations and surgical technique. Int J Oral Maxillofac Surg 2009;38(12):1316–9.

24. Barton FE, Zilmer ME. The cervicofacial flap in cheek reconstruction: anatomic and clinical observations. Presented at the annual meeting of the American Society of Plastic and Reconstructive Surgeons. Honolulu, Hawaii, October 1982.

25. Whetzel TP, Stevenson TR. The contribution of the SMAS to the blood supply in the lateral face lift flap. Plast Reconstr Surg 1997;100(Suppl 1):1011–8.

26. Jacono AA, Rousso JJ, Lavin TJ. Comparing rates of distal edge necrosis in deep-plane vs subcutaneous cervicofacial rotation-advancement flaps for facial cutaneous Mohs defects. JAMA Facial Plast Surg 2014;16(1):31.

27. Boyette JR, Vural E. Cervicofacial advancement-rotation flap in midface reconstruction: forward or reverse? Otolaryngol Head Neck Surg 2011;144(2):196–200.

28. Hanasono MM, Lee JC, Yang JS, et al. An algorithmic approach to reconstructive surgery and prosthetic rehabilitation after orbital exenteration. Plast Reconstr Surg 2009;123(1):98–105.

29. Desciak EB, Eliezri YD. Surgical pearl: temporary suspension suture (frost suture) to help prevent ectropion after infraorbital reconstruction. J Am Acad Dermatol 2003;49(6):1107–8.

30. Rapstine ED, Knaus WJ, Thornton JF. Simplifying cheek reconstruction. Plast Reconstr Surg 2012;129(6):1291–9.

31. Haddock NT, Zide BM. Deep-plane angle rotation flap for reconstruction of perioral lesions. Ann Plast Surg 2011;67(6):594–6.

32. Longaker MT, Glat PM, Zide BM. Deep-plane cervicofacial "hike": anatomic basis with dog-ear blepharoplasty. Plast Reconstr Surg 1997;99(1):16–21.

33. Becker FF, Langford FP. Deep-plane cervicofacial flap for reconstruction of large cheek defects. Arch Otolaryngol Head Neck Surg 1996;122(9):997–9.

34. Tan ST, Mackinnon CA. Deep plane cervicofacial flap: a useful and versatile technique in head and neck surgery. Head Neck 2006;28(1):46–55.

35. Hamra ST. Composite rhytidectomy. Plast Reconstr Surg 1992;90(1):1–13.

36. Austen WG, Parrett BM, Taghinia A, et al. The subcutaneous cervicofacial flap revisited. Ann Plast Surg 2009;62(2):149–53.

37. Cook TA, Israel JM, Wang TD, et al. Cervical rotation flaps for midface resurfacing. Arch Otolaryngol Head Neck Surg 1991;117(1):77–82.

38. Ebrahimi A, Nejadsarvari N. Experience with cervicofacial flap in cheek reconstruction. J Craniofac Surg 2013;24(4):E372–4.

Paramedian Forehead Flap

Ryan J. Smart, DMD, MD, Melvyn S. Yeoh, DMD, MD*, D. David Kim, DMD, MD

KEYWORDS

- Paramedian forehead flap • Forehead flap • Local facial flap • Nasal reconstruction
- Midface reconstruction

KEY POINTS

- The paramedian forehead flap (PMFF) is well suited for reconstructing complex defects of the nose and nasal tip.
- The flap produces an excellent tissue color and texture match for nasal reconstruction.
- The flap is an interpolated axial flap based primarily off the supratrochlear artery. Collateral arteries include the dorsal nasal branch of the angular artery and supraorbital artery. Given such a rich blood supply, this is a reliable and durable flap.
- The pedicle can be narrow allowing primary closure of the donor site inferiorly. Superiorly, when larger areas of tissue are harvested, the surgical site can be left to heal by secondary intention that usually produces a cosmetically acceptable scar.
- Disadvantages include conspicuous donor site, thick flap when used for nasal reconstruction, and requirement for a multistage procedure.
- Complications include poor donor site healing, flap necrosis and hematoma formation, residual nasal deformity, impaired nasal function, and unaesthetic outcome.

INTRODUCTION

Regional flaps to reconstruct nasal structures have been described as early as 600 BC. The origins of the forehead flap for nasal reconstruction can be traced to the forehead rhinoplasty, Indian method, performed by the Khangiara family of India since AD 1400. This classic Indian forehead flap rhinoplasty was popularized in the United States by Kazanjian in the 1930s. Kazanjian had described a vertical flap from the forehead midline supplied by paired supratrochlear vessels. Incisions were made from the hairline to the area above the nasofrontal angle. This flap was then elevated and rotated 180° at the level of the eyebrows to allow for inset into the nasal areas. The Kazanjian-described flap was limited in its reach to the inferior portions of the nasal structure such as the columella. To increase the reach of the flap, subsequent surgeons have tried to modify the length of the incisions to lower the arch of rotation. But it was Millard who demonstrated that bilateral supratrochlear artery pedicles were not essential for flap viability and that central forehead tissue can reliably be transferred on a unilateral paramedian blood supply, which lowered the arc of rotation increasing flap length.

Disclosure: The authors have no financial disclosures to report.
Department of Oral and Maxillofacial Surgery/Head and Neck Surgery, Louisiana State University Health Sciences Center, Shreveport, LA, USA
* Corresponding author.
E-mail address: melvynyeoh@gmail.com

Oral Maxillofacial Surg Clin N Am 26 (2014) 401–410
http://dx.doi.org/10.1016/j.coms.2014.05.008
1042-3699/14/$ – see front matter © 2014 Elsevier Inc. All rights reserved.

oralmaxsurgery.theclinics.com

Anatomic studies by McCarthy and colleagues[1] in the 1980s supported Millard's technique and showed that the blood supply to the forehead is from an arcade of vessels supplied by the supratrochlear, infratrochlear, supraorbital, dorsonasal, and angular branches of the facial artery. This robust anastomotic plexus is actually centered on the medial canthal region and can supply a unilaterally based flap even after division of the supratrochlear, supraorbital, and infraorbital vessels. The modern PMFF is perfused by this rich vertically oriented axial blood supply with its arc of rotation located near the medial canthus and has the ability to reach the columella.[2]

Subtle modifications based on specific patient requirements have been described without alteration of this blood supply.[3–5] The PMFF is also commonly used concomitantly with other procedures such as bone and cartilage grafts for total nasal reconstruction.[6–8] Split flaps and adjunctive tissue expansion modifications of the PMFF have also been described.[9–11] This article describes a traditional 2-stage technique and presents the case of a patient with a posttraumatic nasal deformity reconstructed with a PMFF (**Fig. 1**).

INDICATIONS/CONTRAINDICATIONS

Indications and contraindications of the paramedian forehead flap	
Indications	**Contraindications**
• Reconstruction of complex posttraumatic and postablative nasal deformities • Deformity of the nasal-orbital ethmoid complex, medial canthus and radix[11–13] • Reconstruction of the exenterated orbit[14]	• Patients with soft tissue loss or prior surgery or trauma at the donor site • Patients unwilling or unable to tolerate multiple staged operation

TECHNIQUE/PROCEDURE
Preoperative Planning

The preoperative nasal subunit analysis is one of the many elements considered when planning nasal reconstruction with the PMFF.[2,15] The placement of incisions is important when reconstructing facial structures. Ideally, incisions should be placed in natural creases and borders such as between the nasal subunits to minimize the appearance of scars. The sole use of nasal subunit analysis to plan nasal reconstruction has led some surgeons to become overzealous in the removal of healthy tissue, resulting in less esthetic outcomes. In a retrospective review of 1334 nasal reconstruction cases, Rohrich and colleagues[16] cautioned against this overreliance on the subunit principle because it had resulted in the loss of excessive healthy surrounding nasal tissue and the need to reconstruct larger defects. However, the nasal subunit analysis is important because it allows the surgeon to identify what structures have been lost or altered and areas that may require reconstruction. This analysis is only one of the many considerations when determining a patient's reconstructive needs.

In patients with a naturally low anterior hairline or a prominent widow's peak, gaining adequate flap length can be an issue. In these cases, the surgeon may consider extending the incision for the pedicle through the eyebrow toward the level of the superior medial orbital rim and then dissecting the pedicle from the surrounding soft tissues around the supratrochlear artery. But by doing this, the vascular contributions from the supraorbital plexus are decreased, and caution should be exercised in patients at risk for vascular compromise. An alternate method for these patients may be to angle the distal portion of the flap in an oblique manner just inferior to the hairline to increase flap length. If hair-bearing scalp must be incorporated into the flap, depilatory maneuvers can be undertaken, and this is often time consuming, requiring multiple rounds of treatment.

Another method of increasing flap size is through the placement of a tissue expander before flap elevation. Kheradmand and colleagues[9] reported on 48 patients who had a tissue expander placed before forehead flap elevation. The investigators commented that this technique had allowed for better control of the flap thickness, had improved vascular supply to all layers of the flap, had increased the availability of tissue for reconstruction, and had made primary closure of the donor site easier.[9] Opponents to this technique have argued that the placement of tissue expanders causes an extra step and a conspicuous forehead deformity preoperatively.[2] The authors limit the use of the expander to cases in which dual flaps will be elevated and when most of the central forehead tissue is planned for harvest.

When treating patients with vascular compromise such as patients with atherosclerotic

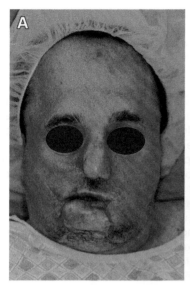
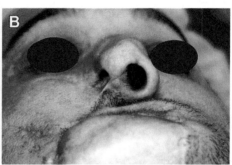

Fig. 1. (*A*, *B*) Frontal and subnasal view of a patient with acquired nasal defect after firearm injury. Note the absence of alar cartilage, deviation of the nasal tip, and stenosis of the right naris.

disease, diabetes, or long-standing tobacco use, surgical delay of the forehead flap is advised. To delay a flap, the dimensions of the defect are determined and marked over the territory of the planned pedicle. The proposed flap edges are then incised to periosteum. In most cases, a few millimeters of the peripheral outline are left intact to ensure that the flap can handle this intervention. These minor tissue connections are then transected before formal flap transfer approximately 3 to 4 weeks later. The rationale of surgical delay is to induce vasodilation by depleting adrenergic factors through severing nearby nerve endings. This reduction in the release of vasoconstrictive metabolites and ischemic condition induces neoangiogenesis improving overall vascularity to the flap's pedicle base after a few weeks.[2,15,17,18] Other reasons to surgically delay a flap can include a significant old scar that lies within the proposed flap territory, a suspect pedicle's main blood supply due to previous injury, unusually complex extensions of the flap, flap design extending across one vascular territory into another, or a patient with history of facial radiation.

Anatomic Considerations

Understanding the vascular anatomy of the supratrochlear artery and supraorbital plexus is paramount to understanding the design of the PMFF. Shumrick and Smith[19] elegantly described this

vascular anatomy based on cadaveric and radiographic studies. The forehead's rich vascular supply consists of the supraorbital plexus that is fed by the dorsal nasal, supratrochlear, and supraorbital arteries. This plexus extends as cephalad as 7 mm superior to the superior orbital rim.[18] The supratrochlear artery was reported by Shumrick and Smith[19] to exit the superior medial orbit 1.7–2.2 cm lateral to the midline with continuation superiorly in a paramedian position approximately 2 cm lateral to the midline.

It is common practice to use a Doppler probe to map out the location of the artery before incision. Ugur and colleagues[20] performed a Doppler imaging study, correlated their findings in live subjects with detailed cadaver dissections, and demonstrated that the supratrochlear artery lies within 3 mm lateral or medial to the medial can thus. The investigators also found that it was located more medially in female subjects.

Vural and colleagues[21] performed a similar study using Doppler imaging in live subjects with cadaver correlation. The investigators found that the supratrochlear artery was localized at the lateral margin of the glabellar frown lines in about 50% of patients and within 3.2 mm lateral to this landmark in the remaining subjects. Even if these anatomic landmarks are to be used, it is still prudent to confirm with the Doppler stethoscope before incision given the ease of use and availability of Doppler units.

As the supratrochelar artery proceeds superiorly, it pierces the orbital septum and lies just over the periosteum as it crosses the supraorbital rim. In this area, it passes between the orbicularis and corrugator muscles. The artery then pierces the frontalis muscle at approximately 1 cm superior to the eyebrow to travel in a subcutaneous plane toward the hairline where it terminates in the subdermal plexus.[19] Some surgeons recommend elevating the frontalis muscle along with the flap to protect the vessel, whereas others have described the safety of elevating a thinner flap while leaving the frontalis muscle intact in order to produce a more tailored flap. By elevating this thinner flap, the surgeon is able to better replicate the thin tissues over the nasal tip.[2,18,19]

SURGICAL PROCEDURE
Surgical Armamentarium

Instrumentation for the forehead flap consists of a Doppler unit with gel, skin marker, cut glove or other sterile material for pattern fabrication, scalpel, periosteal elevators, skin hooks, local anesthetic, and sutures for closure. The authors favor 4-0 Vicryl sutures for deep layer closure and 5-0 nylon sutures for skin closure. The use of a beaver blade in intricate areas around the naris and nasal tip is recommended but not required.[15]

Preoperative Preparation

The PMFF procedure can be performed in the outpatient surgery setting either under intravenous (IV) sedation with local anesthesia or under general anesthesia based on the surgeon's preference and the patient's needs. In general, the patient is positioned in the supine or semireclined position. If placed supine, it is useful to place the patient in reverse Trendelenburg position to facilitate venous drainage of the face to minimize bleeding. If the procedure is completed under general anesthesia, the patient's eyes should be closed and protected with Tegaderm or Steri-Strip (3M Healthcare, Maplewood, MN, USA). The mouth should also be covered, if the patient is intubated, to minimize contamination of the surgical field. When the procedure is done under sedation, the patient should be instructed to keep the eyes closed to prevent injury and a nasal canula should be placed by the mouth for supplemental oxygen. Antibiotics with staphylococcus coverage should be given before incision. The entire nose, cheeks, and forehead should be prepared in a sterile manner before incision.

Using a Doppler and a skin marker, the path of the supratrochlear artery is mapped out. Nasal subunits are also drawn (Fig. 2). A piece of latex glove or sterile template material is then placed over the defect and trimmed to the dimensions required. This template is then rotated from the defect onto the forehead. Care is taken to center the template on the previously marked supratrochlear artery for planning of the incisions over the harvest site. The pedicle portion of the flap can be as narrow as 1.5 cm without compromising the flap. A narrower pedicle allows for an easier primary closure over the inferior portion of the flap. When planning the flap, it is vital to take into consideration the pedicle length required because a template placed too inferiorly can result in an inability to reach the defect.

Once the markings have been placed, local anesthetic with epinephrine can be injected around the planned incision lines for hemostasis. If the procedure is done under IV sedation, care should be taken to also anesthetize the remaining forehead and nasal radix by blocking the infratrochlear, supratrochelar, and supraorbital branches of the ophthalmic branch of the trigeminal nerve.

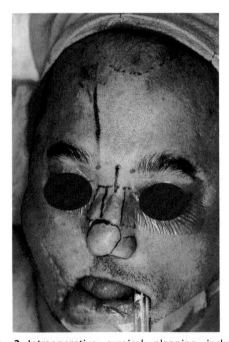

Fig. 2. Intraoperative surgical planning includes marking the supratrochlear artery, the midsagittal point of the nasal radix, the hairline, and the nasal subunits.

Recipient Site Preparation

In preparing the defect site, the margins should be freshened and corners squared off to avoid curvilinear incisions, especially those traveling through esthetic units to avoid depressed or trapdoor scars. In addition, the adjacent skin should be undermined 1 cm around the margin of the defect to facilitate closure.

Flap Harvesting

Next, the flap is incised through skin, subcutaneous tissue muscle, and fascia (**Fig. 3**). The incision is made on the inside of the line drawn using the template to avoid oversizing the flap. Elevation of the flap is then undertaken with blunt dissection in the subfascial plane from superior to inferior leaving periosteum over the frontal bone. Once the corrugator muscle is visualized, it is dissected from the underlying periosteum bluntly to allow greater mobility of the pedicle. On occasion, complete transection of the corrugator muscle is necessary. The pedicle is then freed from the tissues surrounding the superior orbital rim using blunt dissection. If more pedicle length is required, the incision is carried below the level of the eyebrow. This incision is made through skin, and the subcutaneous tissues are dissected gently using a blunt instrument. After harvesting the flap, hemostasis is achieved around the borders of the flap and the flap is covered with a moistened sponge if insetting is delayed.

Alternatively, Ullmann and colleagues[22] describe a novel harvest technique whereby a subcutaneous forehead lift approach is performed. The investigators had noted that the advantages of this technique included excellent direct visualization of the supratrochlear vessels that resulted in an ability to design a thinner flap. Larger harvest site defects were also found to be easier to close primarily with this technique. Instead of the initial incision being around the marked pattern of the flap, they start with a hairline incision and dissect the entire forehead in the subcutaneous plane leaving the frontalis muscle in place. The supratrochlear vessels are then visualized. The entire forehead skin is then turned onto the nasal defect, and the flap is designed to the specifics of the defect being reconstructed based over one of the visualized supratrochlear vessels. The donor site is then closed through rotation and advancement of the 2 remaining lateral forehead flaps toward the midline.

Flap Insertion

During flap inset, the harvested forehead flap is rotated into position over the nasal defect (**Fig. 4**). The distal aspect of the flap can be tailored to the desired thickness. The frontalis muscle and most of the subcutaneous fat can be safely removed from the distal aspect of the flap to achieve this. The flap is then secured in place with 5-0 nylon sutures for precise approximation of the skin edges. If the naris is involved in full-thickness defects, it is useful to place a nasal trumpet to assist in maintaining patency of the nasal passage (**Fig. 5**).

Closing

In order to close the donor site, the forehead is undermined in the subfascial plane from the anterior margin of the temporalis muscles bilaterally. Occasionally, scoring the galea vertically 2 to 3 cm apart can facilitate a large closure (**Fig. 6**). Releasing incisions along the hairline are avoided because this can lead to anesthesia of the anterior scalp, which can be bothersome

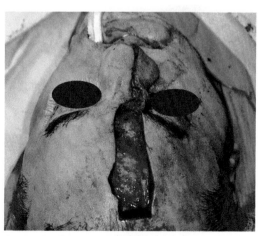

Fig. 4. The flap is rotated 180° along its pedicle and inset to the nasal defect.

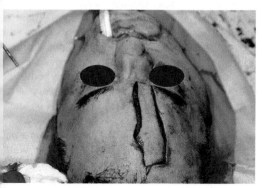

Fig. 3. Incision of the flap before rotation and inset.

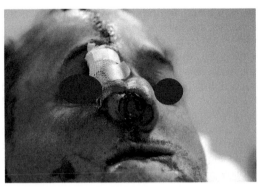

Fig. 5. For full-thickness defects, a nasal trumpet should be used to stent open the naris to prevent collapse.

for patients.[1] In large defects in which primary closure may not be possible, it has been well described that leaving these wounds to heal by secondary intention is a safe and cosmetically acceptable approach.

Montgomery and colleagues[23] described a case in which they used a frontalis muscle flap and full-thickness skin graft to close a large donor site in a patient who underwent nasal reconstruction with a PMFF. The investigators describe rotating the contralateral frontalis muscle into the flap harvest site defect and then using a full-thickness skin graft to cover the muscle.[23]

Second Stage Procedure

Most investigators advocate a period of 3 weeks before division of the pedicle. Somoano and colleagues[24] performed a retrospective review of cases at their institution and found 27 patients

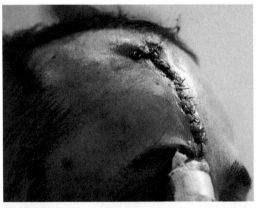

Fig. 6. Often it is possible to obtain primary closure of the forehead donor site with sufficient subfascial undermining of the forehead.

who had undergone division of the pedicle at 1 week. This cohort included patients with history of tobacco use, diabetes, and concomitant cartilage graft use. None of these patients had flap necrosis or tissue loss.[24] Single-stage techniques have also been described in the literature. In the single-stage technique, the flap is de-epithelialized and tunneled under the skin at the radix. The flap is then inset, thus negating the need for a second stage.[25,26]

In those cases requiring pedicle separation, some investigators advocate performing indocyanine green (IC green) angiography to assess distal flap perfusion before division of the pedicle.[27,28] Yeoh and colleagues[29] have previously described the technique for IC green angiography.

Once the flap is deemed viable, the pedicle can be divided under local anesthesia. The pedicle is divided at the superior margin of the defect. The surrounding skin edges are trimmed and undermined to facilitate closure. If further thinning of the flap is necessary, the cephalic portion of the flap and native tissue can be incised and the flap elevated to allow access for thinning. At the base of the pedicle, the interbrow skin is undermined and any scar tissue removed to allow the base of the pedicle to be returned to its initial position. Undermining the adjacent tissue allows release of any contracture and facilitates accurate and equal restoration of brow position and interbrow width. A bolster can then be applied to ensure adherence of the tissue to the underlying nasal framework.

POSTOPERATIVE CARE

After completion of flap inset, the raw surfaces of the flap are cauterized to minimize postoperative bleeding. Wound care consisting of gentle cleansing with warm soap and water and application of topical antimicrobial agents is advised. Debris and crusting are kept at a minimum through meticulous suture line care with dilute hydrogen peroxide. Occasionally, patients must be admitted to the hospital for management of pain and postoperative nausea; however, the procedure itself does not require hospitalization. Although a benefit has not been proven in the literature, Schreiber and Mobley[15] advocate the use of topical nitroglycerin paste every 4 to 6 hours for flaps showing signs of vascular compromise.[15]

After division of the pedicle, the patient is again advised to clean the wound gently with warm soap and water and apply topical antimicrobial ointment to the suture lines twice daily. Crusting and debris are to be kept to a minimum with dilute peroxide. Sutures are removed at 7 days. The patients are advised to avoid sun exposure for 6 months postoperatively to avoid postinflammatory hyperpigmentation. Any further revision procedures are delayed for at least 4 months to allow contracture, scar maturation, and complete wound healing.

ADDITIONAL CONSIDERATIONS

The PMFF can be used in pediatric nasal reconstruction but with some key difference kept in mind. First, the age of the child is important. A child begins to become self-conscious by the age of 5; therefore, restoration closest to normal nasal esthetics is important by this age. Unlike the ear that has fully developed subunits at birth, the nose undergoes developmental changes throughout childhood up to the age of 12 in females and 16 in males. Based on these anatomic differences, Giugliano and colleagues[30] recommend a modified subunit analysis consisting of 3 subunits being the tip, dorsum, and ala. In addition, flap design may need to be cross-forehead or oblique to compensate for the shorter forehead length in pediatric patients.[30] With respect to function, significant alteration in nasal form can result in external valve collapse and stenosis; therefore, all deforming forces on the nose should be thoroughly released and the nose should be carefully reconstructed.[31] An approach to reconstruction after nasal growth has completed is not recommended based on these functional, psychosocial, and esthetic requirements. When reconstructing structural elements, nasal septal cartilage should not be used as a graft donor site because it plays a role in midface growth and development. Rather, conchal or costochondral cartilage grafts should be used.

Nasal defects often consist of multiple tissue layers. All 3 layers of the nose, the external skin, intermediate cartilaginous or bony framework, and internal lining, frequently require reconstruction. When using a PMFF, a plan for reconstruction of all missing layers should be taken into consideration. Various techniques to reconstruct the nasal internal lining have been described, including the turnover skin flap, ipsilateral mucoperichondrial flap, and septal hinge flap.[5,8]

Use of the PMFF for the nose's inner lining reconstruction has been reported by the Brazilian surgeon Roberto Farina. Farina describes tunneling the PMFF under the glabellar skin to be inset as the nasal internal lining. Parikh and colleagues[7] developed a modification to the

Farina method or frontal flap method. These investigators' modification involves using a rhinoplasty approach to gain exposure to the nose for flap inset. Moyer[10] also described a case in which staged bilateral PMFFs were used to reconstruct a near-total nasal defect. The internal lining was first reconstructed and then the external surface of the nose.[10] Potter and colleagues[6] published a series of 9 patients in which a PMFF with a distal pericranial extension was designed. The pericranium was folded into the nasal vestibule to recreate the septal and vestibular lining tissue. This procedure also allowed primary placement of cartilage and bone grafts.

POSSIBLE COMPLICATIONS AND MANAGEMENT

In a recent retrospective review of patients older than 75 years, median age 81 years, who had undergone PMFF reconstruction of nasal defects, Kendler and colleagues[32] identified 28 patients and reported 7 complications (25%). These complications included epidermal necrosis in 2 patients, bleeding in 1 patient, hair on the flap in 1 patient, alar rim notching in 1 patient, and infection-related complications in 2 patients. Notably, many of these patients, in their advanced age, had multiple medical comorbidities and some were on anticoagulant medications. Paddack and colleagues[33] published a retrospective review of 107 patients who underwent PMFF or nasolabial flap reconstruction of nasal defects. The investigators reported an overall 6% failure rate in forehead flaps but did not find any statistically significant predictors of flap failure.[33] In a brief communication by Riggio,[34] a case of flap congestion and necrosis is described in which the patient had undergone bilateral neck dissection at the time of reconstruction using a PMFF. This patient had venous congestion of the flap. The investigator comments that the neck dissection may have impaired venous drainage and that given the rich vascular inflow to the flap, congestion ensued resulting in failure.[34]

Overall, the complication rate for PMFF is low. Flap necrosis may be avoidable in at-risk patients by taking the aforementioned precautions in design of the flap and use of surgical delay. Poor esthetic outcomes, especially with regard to the thin tissues of the nasal tip, can be avoided by proper tissue thinning and tailoring and appropriate use of cartilage and bone grafts for construction of the underlying framework of the nose.

CLINICAL RESULTS IN THE LITERATURE

Outcomes of the paramedian forehead flaps and summary of key principles discussed in recent literature

Study	Citation	Key Points and Findings
Retrospective chart review of patients who underwent PMFF to identify treatment failures and determine contributing factors	Paddack et al,[33] 2012	• 82 of the patients underwent 2-stage PMFF repair • 5 failed, 3 were full-thickness repairs • Use of cartilage grafts did not increase risk of failure • No single comorbidity was noted to have a statistically significant effect on failure rates

Study assessed the esthetic and functional outcomes and complications of FHF in elderly patients with nonmelanoma skin cancer	Kendler et al,[32] 2014	• 28 patients
		• Median age: 81 y (range, 75–95 y)
		  ○ Average defect size was 11 cm² (5–30 cm²)
		  ○ Cartilage grafts were used in 4 patients (14%)
		  ○ Average time to division: 25 d (17–45)
		• 7 treatment-related complications
		  ○ Infectious causes (2)
		  ○ Epidermal necrotic tissue (2)
		  ○ Bleeding (1)
		  ○ Hair on the flap (1)
		  ○ Alar rim notching (1)

Retrospective analysis on 1334 patients who underwent nasal reconstruction after Mohs histographic excisions. Recorded variables included number of operations per patient, locations of defects, and complications	Rohrich et al,[16] 2004	• 1.9% tumor recurrence rate was documented
		• 81% of reconstructions were completed in 3 or fewer stages
		  ○ 75% were 2-staged procedures
		• 1.2% revision rate was noted
		  ○ 13 partial flap necroses required revision
		  ○ 3 patients experienced dehiscence at the donor site
		• Investigators describe a preferred philosophy of reconstruction based on their experience:
		  ○ Maximal conservation of native tissue is advised
		  ○ Reconstruction of the defect, not the subunit, is advised
		  ○ Good contour is the esthetic end point
		  ○ Complementary ablative procedures enhance end result
		  ○ Primary defatting improves contour and reduces revisions
		  ○ Use of axial pattern flaps is preferred

The purpose of this article is to review the authors' experience with the FHF for nasal reconstruction in 10 children under the age of 10 during a 10-year period.	Giugliano et al,[30] 2004	• 10 patients
		  ○ 1 patient lost to follow-up, average follow-up 4.5 y
		• Predefined cosmetic grading system (0 = excellent to 15 = poor)
		  ○ Average score: 5.3
		• Based on results, investigators developed the following tenets of PMFF in children:
		  ○ 3 nasal subunits should be considered in the developing nose
		  ○ FHF is the best option for entire subunit or full-thickness defect
		  ○ Flap design should be paramedian, oblique, and opposite to avoid low hairline and allow better advancement
		  ○ Septal cartilage grafts should be avoided, ear or costal cartilage should be used
		  ○ Skin grafts, infundibular undermining, turnover, and vestibular mucosal flaps are good options for lining
		  ○ A 3-stage procedure should be used (intermediate thinning and secondary procedures for support/lining)
		  ○ Complete reconstruction before child is school-aged
		  ○ Reconstructed nose grows with the child
		  ○ No final surgery should be planned after age 18 (other than revisions of late complications)

Abbreviation: FHF, forehead flap.

SUMMARY

The PMFF is a versatile flap with a robust vascular supply that is well suited for reconstruction of complex or large nasal defects. Although a 2-stage technique is most common, a single-stage procedure involving tunneling the proximal pedicle and 3-stage procedures involving tissue expansion, vascular delay, and flap tailoring after inset before pedicle division have also been described. The flap is safe in a wide age range of adult patients who have acquired postablative deformities and has been shown to be useful in the pediatric populations as well. This flap remains a critical tool in the armamentarium of reconstructive oral and maxillofacial surgeons.

REFERENCES

1. McCarthy JG, Lorenc ZP, Cutting C, et al. The median forehead flap revisited: the blood supply. Plast Reconstr Surg 1985;76(6):866–9.
2. Baker SR. Interpolated paramedian forehead flaps. In: Baker SR, editor. Local flaps in facial reconstruction. Philadelphia: Mosby Elsevier; 2007. p. 265–312.
3. Angobaldo J, Marks M. Refinements in nasal reconstruction: the cross-paramedian forehead flap. Plast Reconstr Surg 2009;123(1):87–93.
4. Menick FJ. Nasal reconstruction with a forehead flap. Clin Plast Surg 2009;36(3):443–59.
5. Moolenburgh SE, McLennan L, Levendag PC, et al. Nasal reconstruction after malignant tumor resection: an algorithm for treatment. Plast Reconstr Surg 2010;126(1):97–105.
6. Potter JK, Ducic Y, Ellis E 3rd. Extended bilaminar forehead flap with cantilevered bone grafts for reconstruction of full-thickness nasal defects. J Oral Maxillofac Surg 2005;63(4):566–70.
7. Parikh S, Futran ND, Most SP. An alternative method for reconstruction of large intranasal lining defects: the Farina method revisited. Arch Facial Plast Surg 2010;12(5):311–4.
8. Bashir MM, Khan BA, Abbas M, et al. Outcome of modified turn in flaps for the lining with primary cartilage support in nasal reconstruction. J Craniofac Surg 2013;24(2):454–7.
9. Kheradmand AA, Garajei A, Motamedi MH. Nasal reconstruction: experience using tissue expansion and forehead flap. J Oral Maxillofac Surg 2011; 69(5):1478–84.
10. Moyer JS. Reconstruction of extensive nasal defects with staged bilateral paramedian forehead flaps. Ann Plast Surg 2010;65(2):188–92.
11. Onaran Z, Yazici I, Karakaya EI, et al. Simultaneous reconstruction of medial canthal area and both eyelids with a single transverse split forehead island flap. J Craniofac Surg 2011;22(1):363–5.
12. Krishnamurthy A. Split paramedian forehead flap for medial canthal reconstruction. Natl J Maxillofac Surg 2012;3(2):241–2. http://dx.doi.org/10.4103/0975-5950.111399.
13. Price DL, Sherris DA, Bartley GB, et al. Forehead flap periorbital reconstruction. Arch Facial Plast Surg 2004;6(4):222–7.
14. Sharma RK. Supratrochlear artery island paramedian forehead flap for reconstructing the exenterated patient. Orbit 2011;30(3):154–7.
15. Schreiber NT, Mobley SR. Elegant solutions for complex paramedian forehead flap reconstruction. Facial Plast Surg Clin North Am 2011;19(3):465–79.
16. Rohrich RJ, Griffin JR, Ansari M, et al. Nasal reconstruction—beyond aesthetic subunits: a 15-year review of 1334 cases. Plast Reconstr Surg 2004; 114(6):1405–16.
17. Kent DE, Defazio JM. Improving survival of the paramedian forehead flap in patients with excessive tobacco use: the vascular delay. Dermatol Surg 2011;37(9):1362–4.
18. Pawar SS, Kim MM. Updates in forehead flap reconstruction of facial defects. Curr Opin Otolaryngol Head Neck Surg 2013;21(4):384–8.
19. Shumrick KA, Smith TL. The anatomic basis for the design of forehead flaps in nasal reconstruction. Arch Otolaryngol Head Neck Surg 1992;118(4): 373–9.
20. Ugur MB, Savranlar A, Uzun L, et al. A reliable surface landmark for localizing supratrochlear artery: medial can thus. Otolaryngol Head Neck Surg 2008;138(2):162–5.
21. Vural E, Batay F, Key JM. Glabellar frown lines as a reliable landmark for the supratrochlear artery. Otolaryngol Head Neck Surg 2000;123(5):543–6.
22. Ullmann Y, Fodor L, Shoshani O, et al. A novel approach to the use of the paramedian forehead flap for nasal reconstruction. Plast Reconstr Surg 2005;115(5):1372–8.
23. Montgomery J, Mace AT, Cotter C, et al. Frontalis muscle flap: a novel method for donor site closure of an interpolated paramedian forehead flap. J Laryngol Otol 2010;124(4):453–5.
24. Somoano B, Kampp J, Gladstone HB. Accelerated takedown of the paramedian forehead flap at 1 week: indications, technique, and improving patient quality of life. J Am Acad Dermatol 2011;65(1):97–105.
25. Fudem GM, Montilla RD, Vaughn CJ. Single-stage forehead flap in nasal reconstruction. Ann Plast Surg 2010;64(5):645–8.
26. Kishi K, Imanishi N, Shimizu Y, et al. Alternative 1-step nasal reconstruction technique. Arch Facial Plast Surg 2012;14(2):116–21.
27. Woodard CR, Most SP. Intraoperative angiography using laser-assisted indocyanine green imaging to

map perfusion of forehead flaps. Arch Facial Plast Surg 2012;14:263–9.

28. Shah A, Au A. CASE REPORT laser-assisted indocyanine green evaluation of paramedian forehead flap perfusion prior to pedicle division. Eplasty 2013;13:e8.

29. Yeoh MS, Kim DD, Ghali GE. Fluorescence angiography in the assessment of flap perfusion and vitality. Oral Maxillofac Surg Clin North Am 2013;25(1): 61–6, vi.

30. Giugliano C, Andrades PR, Benitez S. Nasal reconstruction with a forehead flap in children younger than 10 years of age. Plast Reconstr Surg 2004; 114(2):316–25.

31. Lee EI, Xue AS, Hollier LH Jr, et al. Ear and nose reconstruction in children. Oral Maxillofac Surg Clin North Am 2012;24(3):397–416.

32. Kendler M, Averbeck M, Wetzig T. Reconstruction of nasal defects with forehead flaps in patients older than 75 years of age. J Eur Acad Dermatol Venereol 2014;28(5):662–6.

33. Paddack AC, Frank RW, Spencer HJ, et al. Outcomes of paramedian forehead and nasolabial interpolation flaps in nasal reconstruction. Arch Otolaryngol Head Neck Surg 2012;138(4):367–71.

34. Riggio E. The hazards of contemporary paramedian forehead flap and neck dissection in smokers. Plast Reconstr Surg 2003;112(1):346–7.

The Supraclavicular Artery Island and Trapezius Myocutaneous Flaps in Head and Neck Reconstruction

Carlos A. Ramirez, DDS, MD[a],*,
Rui P. Fernandes, DMD, MD[b,c]

KEYWORDS

• Supraclavicular artery flap • Trapezius flap • Pedicled flap • Reconstruction

KEY POINTS

- The supraclavicular artery island flap can be readily used to reconstruct defects within the neck, parotid, lateral temporal region, and lower third of the face.
- Benefits of the supraclavicular flap include good color and texture match, an ease of harvest, and minimal donor site morbidity; there is also no significant post-operative monitoring required.
- The trapezius muscle serves as a source for multiple myocutaneous flaps of which most are considered to be salvage flaps among head and neck reconstructive surgeons.
- The major blood supply to both the supraclavicular and trapezius flaps originates from the transverse cervical artery; radical neck dissection that ligates this vessel will render both of these flap nonviable options on the ipsilateral side.

 Video of SCAF FLAP ELEVATION accompanies this article at http://www.oralmaxsurgery.theclinics. com/

The surgical management of head and neck oncologic defects has been revolutionized since the advent of microvascular free tissue autotransplantation. Ablative surgeons, knowing that the reconstructive surgeon can likely harvest a larger flap, are able to resect with wider margins to assure complete removal of the cancer. In certain cases, however, an argument is made against the use of a microvascular reconstruction given the individual patient's medical comorbidities, the availability of vessels in the neck, the extended operative time required for microvascular procedures, the infrastructure required to perform and monitor the microvascular flaps post-operatively, and the surgical expertise needed. In addition, previously operated patients, those with complications secondary to radiotherapy, and those who have failed free flap reconstruction pose a significant

---
[a] Division of Oral and Maxillofacial Surgery, Center for Head and Neck, Maxillofacial & Reconstructive Surgery, St. John Providence Health System, 11900 East 12 Mile Road, Suite 308, Warren, MI 48093, USA; [b] Department of Oral and Maxillofacial Surgery, College of Medicine, University of Florida, 653-1 West Eighth Street, LRC 2nd Floor, Jacksonville, FL 32209, USA; [c] Division of Surgical Oncology, Department of Surgery, College of Medicine, University of Florida, 653-1 West Eighth Street, LRC 2nd Floor, Jacksonville, FL 32209, USA
* Corresponding author.
E-mail address: carlos.ramirez@stjohn.org

Oral Maxillofacial Surg Clin N Am 26 (2014) 411–420
http://dx.doi.org/10.1016/j.coms.2014.05.009
1042-3699/14/$ – see front matter © 2014 Elsevier Inc. All rights reserved.

reconstructive challenge to the surgeon. It is for these cases that the reconstructive surgeon must have local and regional flaps available within their armamentarium to fulfill the reconstructive needs of the patient. The supraclavicular artery island flap and the trapezius myocutaneous flap, either alone or in combination, are reliably used to reconstruct a wide array of head and neck defects and are pivotal to the arsenal of any reconstructive surgeon.

SUPRACLAVICULAR ARTERY ISLAND FLAP
History

In 1842, Mütter first described the shoulder flap, which at that time was harvested as a random patterned flap.[1] In 1903, Toldt, an anatomist, illustrated and named the *arteria cervicalis superficialis*, which originated from the thyrocervical trunk and exited between the sternocleidomastoid and the trapezius muscles. Kazanjian and Converse, in 1949, described this flap as the "*in charretera*" or acromial flap and showed its first clinical utility in burn scar contracture resurfacing. *Charretera* describes the region over the shoulders on which honors are bestowed on military personnel.[2] Mathes and Vasconez renamed this flap the cervicohumeral flap in 1978 based on their anatomic studies.[3] Lamberty, in 1979 and again with Cormack in 1983, described the supraclavicular fasciocutaneous island flap.[4] During the 1980s, with concerns being raised regarding distal flap necrosis and as the popularity of the pectoralis major flap increased, this flap fell out of favor with head and neck reconstructive surgeons. It was not until the late 1990s when Pallua and colleagues[5] performed further anatomic studies and "rediscovered" the supraclavicular artery island flap and its use in releasing post-burn mentosternal contractures in a reliable fashion. Di Benedetto, in 2004, described the supraclavicular fascial island flap where a fascial pedicle was maintained to ensure protection of the vessels from excessive stretch or compression preventing distal flap tip necrosis.[6] Saint-Cyr and Chiu, in 2010, published their study on the vascular anatomy and perfusion of the supraclavicular flap and noted direct linking vessels between perforators and recurrent flow by means of the subdermal plexus. This study explained how perfusion is maintained to the distal periphery of the flap, further attesting to the reliability of the vascular pedicle.[7]

Anatomy

Originating from the thyrocervical trunk, the transverse cervical artery gives rise to the supraclavicular artery in 93% of cases. In the remaining 7% of cases, the supraclavicular artery can arise from the suprascapular artery. Numerous anatomic studies have confirmed the presence of multiple skin perforators and the presence of interperforator flow between adjacent perforators. The artery is localized 8 cm lateral to the sternoclavicular joint, 3 cm superior to the clavicle, and 2 cm posterior to the sternocleidomastoid. The artery is reported to be present in 80% to 100% of individuals. The vessel diameter averages 1.0 to 1.5 mm at its origin. If the vessel at its origin is less than 1 mm in diameter, the surface area of flap perfusion can be diminished. The length of the vessel can vary from 1 to 7 cm. One to two venae comitantes run with the supraclavicular artery, and they drain into the transverse cervical vein. The diameter of the transverse cervical vein at its origin is 2.5 mm.[8] The sensory nerve supply arises from the supraclavicular nerves (C3, C4).[9] A flap measuring up to 12 cm × 35 cm can be harvested; however, widths beyond 7 cm will likely need additional grafting to close.

Indications

The supraclavicular artery island flap has been used in vessel-depleted necks secondary to neck dissections or radiation therapy.[10] With regards to neck dissections, as long as the thyrocervical trunk in level V has not been injured, the ipsilateral flap can still be harvested. Patients with significant medical comorbidities that are not suitable candidates for microvascular reconstruction are able to tolerate the harvest and inset of this regional flap well. The flap is used for partial or circumferential pharyngoesophageal reconstruction following oncologic resection.[11] Facial contour defects secondary to parotidectomy, hemifacial atrophy, or hemifacial microsomia, as well as defects along the infratemporal and lateral skull base, may also benefit from its use.[12,13] It can also be used for anterior chest wall defect reconstruction to obliterate dead space and allow coverage of areas of compromised vascularity.[14] In addition, the flap is used for post-burn neck scar contracture release and soft tissue ablation repair of the lip, chin, and cheek and oropharynx (**Boxes 1** and **2**).[15]

IMAGING

Although not absolutely necessary, preoperative 3D computed tomography angiography (CTA) is obtained to determine the patency of the vascular pedicle. Most importantly, open communication between the ablative and reconstructive surgeon must be had, especially if level V of the neck is to be dissected during surgery (**Figs. 1** and **2**).

Box 1
Supraclavicular artery island flap advantages

- Increased color and texture match with the skin of the face
- Thin and pliable
- Vascularized
- Sensate and hairless
- Low donor site morbidity
- Ease of harvest
- Decreased operative time versus microvascular surgery

Technique

1. Place the patient in the supine position with a shoulder bump under the ipsilateral donor site to improve exposure. If the ipsilateral neck has been radiated or operated on, then the contralateral neck should be used to avoid dissection through scar tissue.
2. Map the course of the supraclavicular artery within the triangular fossa bordered by the sternocleidomastoid muscle, trapezius muscle, and clavicle. The origin of the supraclavicular artery is within a triangle formed by the sternocleidomastoid muscle, the medial third of the clavicle, and the external jugular vein.
3. An elliptical skin paddle is marked out from the root of the neck to the middeltoid muscle. A skin paddle width of up to 7 cm and length of up to 20 cm can be harvested without additional skin grafting.
4. Dissection begins from the distal end and proceeds in a proximal direction within a subfascial plane with the electrocautery. This dissection is performed quickly up until the proximal one-third of the flap. At this point, bipolar forceps should be used for the remainder of the pedicle dissection. Handheld Doppler or transillumination is used to confirm the pedicle location. The external jugular vein does run through the

Box 2
Supraclavicular artery island flap disadvantages

- Anatomic variations of the supraclavicular artery
- Not suitable for large volume defects without expansion
- Donor site scar on shoulder in women
- Potential distal flap necrosis

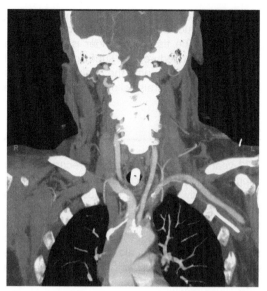

Fig. 1. Computed tomography angiography (CTA) neck: demonstrating patency of thyrocervical trunk.

flap and can be sacrificed, if necessary, to increase the arc of rotation.

Once the pedicle has been identified, the proximal skin island is divided, and the pedicle skeletonized (if necessary) to allow for an increased arc of rotation up to 180° (Video 1; available online at http://www.oralmaxsurgery.theclinics.com/).

5. The flap can be inset with minimal tension using 3-0 Vicryl and 4-0 Prolene sutures to perform the layered closure. Portions of the flap can be deepithelialized to allow for subplatysmal tunneling of the flap, if necessary.
6. The donor site is closed after adequate undermining in a two-layered fashion, and a quarter-inch Penrose drain can be placed.

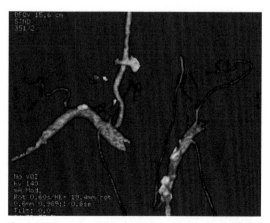

Fig. 2. CTA neck: visible branches of the thyrocervical trunk.

7. Tissue expanders have been used with this flap to reconstruct extensive burns or oncologic resections. The tissue expander is placed in a separate procedure in a subfascial plane and expanded serially until the desired flap size is obtained. This will also allow for primary closure of the donor site.

Case Example

Case #1

A 72-year-old man presented with recurrence of a supraglottic squamous cell carcinoma after being treated initially 20 years previously by radiation therapy. He underwent total laryngectomy with near total circumferential pharyngectomy, bilateral neck dissections, and radial forearm free flap reconstruction. Subsequent to the procedure, the anterior neck skin dehisced and the radial forearm flap vascular pedicle became exposed. The patient was then taken to the operation theatre for coverage of the anterior neck with a supraclavicular flap (**Figs. 3–5**).

Case #2

A 62-year-old woman presented with squamous cell carcinoma of the floor of mouth, tongue, mandible, and overlying chin skin. Patient underwent tracheostomy, composite resection with bilateral neck dissections, and osteocutaneous fibula free flap reconstruction. The distal 10% of the skin paddle dehisced, the residual skin paddle overlying the chin was deepithelialized and a supraclavicular flap was elevated to recontour the chin (**Figs. 6 and 7**).

Case #3

A 55-year-old uncontrolled diabetic man presented for reconstruction following segmental mandibulectomy secondary to osteomyelitis. Patient underwent anterior iliac crest bone graft

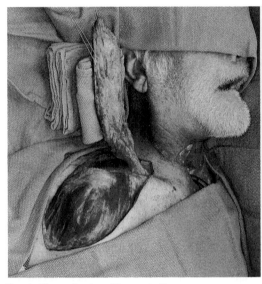

Fig. 4. Flap raised and harvest site.

reconstruction with supraclavicular flap for intraoral lining due to severe scar formation and a lack of vestibular height. The supraclavicular flap was deepithelialized along the portion tunneled through the neck, and the residual skin paddle was inset intraorally (**Figs. 8 and 9**).

Complications

Potential complications, like other flaps, include the risk of complete flap loss, partial flap loss (distal tip), cellulitis (**Fig. 10**), donor site wound dehiscence, or a widened scar at the donor site. With the different potential reconstructions being undertaken with this flap, the complications will depend on the defect being reconstructed. Most complications will arise during pharyngeal reconstruction, with fistula formation being the most

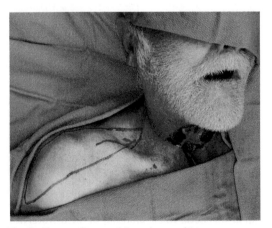

Fig. 3. Flap outline and Doppler markings.

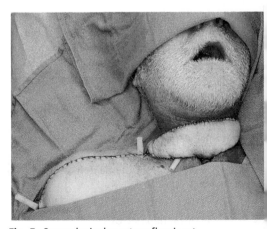

Fig. 5. Supraclavicular artery flap inset.

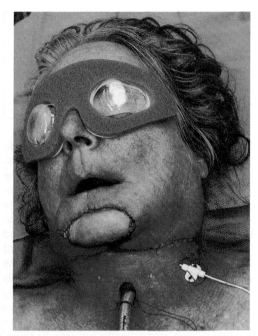

Fig. 6. Distal skin paddle dehiscence fibula flap skin paddle.

common complication encountered. Conservative management of the fistula (diversion and nothing by mouth status) has been reported to allow for healing without further surgical intervention.[16]

Discussion

The supraclavicular flap is readily used to reconstruct tumor-related defects or areas affected by scar contracture within the neck and lower third of the face. It has a reliable vascular pedicle that will allow its utility in medically compromised patients with obesity, diabetes, malnutrition, or chronic smoking and in those with vessel-depleted necks secondary to surgery or radiation therapy. Flap survival is comparable to other

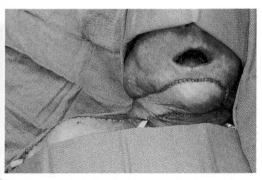

Fig. 7. Supraclavicular flap inset with primary closure of the harvest site.

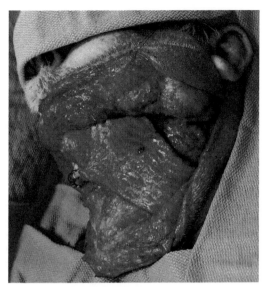

Fig. 8. Supraclavicular flap: tunneled and deepithelialized.

pedicled or free flaps. The benefit being that a microvascular anastomosis is not performed and there is no significant post-operative monitoring required. This flap has solidified a place within head and neck reconstruction and, given its ease of harvest and lack of microsurgical expertise required, should be incorporated into the arsenal of reconstructive oral and maxillofacial surgeons.

TRAPEZIUS MYOCUTANEOUS FLAP
History

The trapezius muscle serves as a source for multiple variations of myocutaneous flaps of which most are considered to be salvage flaps among head and neck reconstructive surgeons. The flaps include the superior trapezius, the lateral island trapezius, the vertical trapezius, the lower island trapezius, and the extended vertical lower trapezius island flap. Conley, in 1972, described the superior trapezius flap, based on the paraspinous perforating branches of the posterior intercostal vessels.[17] Panje and Demergasso described the

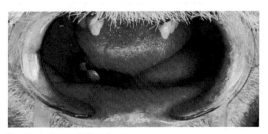

Fig. 9. Intraoral flap inset.

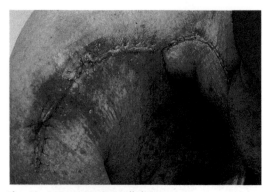

Fig. 10. Post-operative cellulitis.

lateral island trapezius flap, based on the transverse cervical vessels.[18,19] Mathes and Nahai described the vertical trapezius myocutanous flap in 1979.[20] Baek and colleagues[21] described the lower island flap, based on the transverse cervical vessels, in 1980. The lower island vertical trapezius flap is routinely the first choice for resurfacing lateral neck and lateral skull defects; however, after ipsilateral radical neck dissection, the absence of the transverse cervical vessels may preclude its use. The superior trapezius myocutaneous flap is especially useful in lateral neck reconstruction after prior radical neck dissection for coverage of exposed major neck vessels and wound breakdown following radiotherapy. The literature supports the superior trapezius as the most reliable of the flap variants based on the "choke" vessel angiosome concept of Taylor and Palmer.[22] The superior trapezius and lower island (vertical) variants will be discussed.

Anatomy

The trapezius muscle is a large, thin, triangular muscle that originates from the superior nuchal line and external occipital protuberance, the ligamentum nuchae, the seventh cervical vertebra and all the thoracic vertebrae. The occipital and upper cervical fibers of the muscle insert into the posterior border of the lateral one-third of the

clavicle. The lower cervical and upper thoracic fibers insert on the medial border of the acromion and along the upper border of the crest of the spine of the scapula. The trapezius aids in suspending and stabilizing the shoulder girdle as well as raising and rotating the shoulder. The muscle is innervated by the spinal accessory nerve and from direct branches of the ventral rami of the third and fourth cervical nerves. The blood supply to the trapezius muscle and overlying skin is primarily from the superficial and deep descending branches of the transverse cervical artery, as well as the occipital artery. The superficial descending branch arises directly from the thyrocervical trunk in 75% to 80% of cases and is what is known as the transverse cervical artery.[23] The dorsal scapular artery arises from the subclavian artery in 75% of cases; however, in 25% of cases, it arises from the transverse cervical artery, and in these cases, the vessel is named the deep descending branch of the transverse cervical artery, and the junction of the 2 descending branches is the cervicodorsal trunk. The transverse cervical artery enters the trapezius muscle at the base of the neck and descends vertically along the deep surface of the trapezius. The dorsal scapular artery runs under the levator muscle, and its major branch penetrates between the rhomboid muscles and descends along the deep surface of the trapezius to supply the lower third of the trapezius. Additional blood supply is derived from the paraspinous muscle perforating branches of the inferior cervical and thoracic posterior intercostal arteries (**Boxes 3–6**).

Box 4
Superior trapezius flap disadvantages

- Limited arc of rotation and reach, limited to ipsilateral neck defects because it cannot extend beyond the midline
- May require donor site skin graft

Box 3
Superior trapezius flap advantages

- Can be used after ipsilateral neck dissection
- No further functional loss after denervation following radical neck dissection
- Has a superiorly based pedicle, reducing the problem of gravitational pull on the recipient bed

---

Box 5
Lower island (vertical) trapezius flap advantages

- Long arc of rotation
- Long, thin pedicle allows for easy transfer
- Thinner and more pliable
- Adequate soft tissue bulk to cover large soft tissue defects
- Hairless nature of the skin can be advantageous in oral cavity reconstruction

Imaging

Although not absolutely necessary, pre-operative 3D CTA can be obtained to determine the patency of the vascular pedicle. Most importantly, open communication between the ablative and reconstructive surgeon must be had, especially if level V of the neck is to be dissected during surgery (**Fig. 11**).

Technique

Superior trapezius

1. Place patient in the supine or modified lateral decubitus position with exposure of the shoulder to midline of the back.[24]
2. The anterior limb of incision is placed along the anterior border of the trapezius.

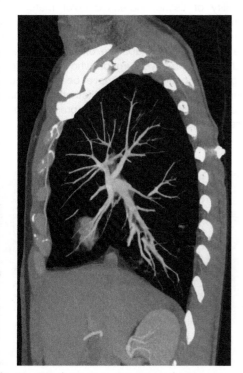

Fig. 11. CTA chest: transverse cervical artery.

3. The posterior horizontal limb is drawn parallel to the anterior horizontal limb, at the level of or above the scapular spine.
4. The lateral aspect of the flap is elevated in a subfascial plane of the deltoid.
5. At the acromion, the trapezius is sharply incised and elevated off its bony insertions down to the supraspinatus muscles.
6. The arc of rotation can be increased by dividing the transverse cervical vessels, if they are present, or by making a superior back cut along the posterior incision.
7. The donor site is closed primarily, after wide undermining, with 2-0 Vicryl suture in the deep layer and 3-0 Prolene suture along the skin. If the donor site cannot be closed primarily, a split thickness skin graft can be harvested and inset.

Vertical trapezius

1. Pre-operative mapping of the transverse cervical vessels should be completed.
2. Place the patient in the lateral decubitus position.
3. The flap should be designed along the route of the transverse cervical artery. The long axis of the flap is centered between the vertebral column and the medial border of the scapula. The medial border of the flap is marked 1 to 2 cm lateral to the spinal processes.
4. The width of the flap should not exceed 8 cm so as to be able to close the defect primarily.
5. The pivot point of the flap is accepted as the level of the scapular spine to preserve the superior fibers of the trapezius muscle. The length of the flap is usually an average of 34 cm (minimum 5 × 30 cm, maximum 7 × 38 cm).
6. Flap elevation begins at the midpoint of the flap along the medial border. Once the trapezius muscle fibers are identified and the medial vertebral insertions are transected, the distal and proximal dissection of the muscle and overlying skin is completed. The transverse cervical artery and vein are identified within the deep fascia on the undersurface of the muscle. Once the vessels have been identified and preserved, the lateral border of the flap can be elevated. Approximately 10 to 13 cm of flap may extend beyond the caudal end of the trapezius muscle.
7. Care should be taken not to violate the underlying latissimus dorsi and rhomboid muscles. Note: at the transition between the rhomboid major and minor, the dorsal scapular artery is

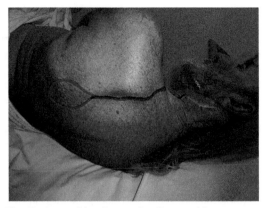

Fig. 12. Lower island trapezius flap marking.

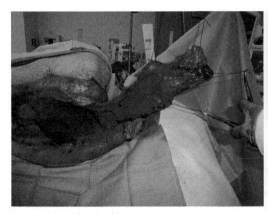

Fig. 14. Flap elevated.

identified lateral to the transverse cervical artery and is divided. This will allow release of the flap and cranial dissection.

8. Dissection cranially ends at the level of the scapular spine (second thoracic vertebrae) to preserve the lateral attachment of the trapezius to the scapular spine and acromion to prevent shoulder droop and weakness. Function is sacrificed by continuing the dissection to the point of entrance of the transverse cervical artery above the levator to increase pedicle length.
9. The donor area is closed primarily in a layered fashion.

Lower island (vertical) trapezius island

1. Dissection as described earlier.[25]
2. The skin island that can be harvested is 8 to 12 cm in length and 5 to 7 cm in width.
3. Once dissection is taken to the pivot point, as described earlier, a subcutaneous tunnel is created and the flap transferred to cover craniomaxillofacial defects.

Case Example

A 57-year-old man presented with hardware exposure following segmental resection and ipsilateral neck dissection in which the transverse cervical artery was preserved. The patient underwent hardware removal with overlying skin excision and was reconstructed with a lower island (vertical) trapezius flap (**Figs. 12–16**).

Discussion

Although the trapezius system of flaps are considered salvage flaps, they do offer significant advantages to the reconstructive surgeon: increased pliability of tissue, increased color match and texture, decreased operating time, and decreased complication rates compared with microvascular free flaps.[26] These flaps are of significant value to the reconstructive surgeon who must perform surgery on patients who have been previously operated, have undergone radiotherapy, or have recurrence of disease in the presence of a vessel-depleted neck.

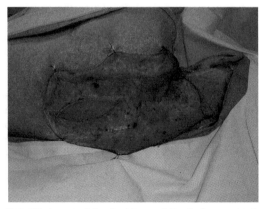

Fig. 13. Lower island skin paddle before muscle division.

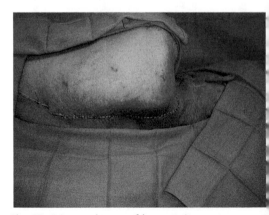

Fig. 15. Primary closure of harvest site.

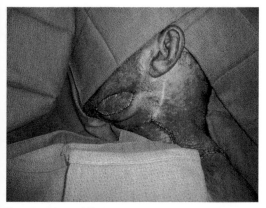

Fig. 16. Skin paddle inset.

SUPPLEMENTARY DATA

Supplementary data related to this article can be found online at http://dx.doi.org/10.1016/j.coms. 2014.05.009.

REFERENCES

1. Mutter T. Case of deformity from Burns relieved by operation. Am J Med Sci 1842;4:66–80.

2. Kazanjian VH, Converse JM. The surgical treatment of facial injuries. Baltimore (MD): Williams & Wilkins; 1949.

3. Mathes SJ, Vasconez LO. The cervico-humeral flap. Plast Reconstr Surg 1978;61:7–12.

4. Lamberty BG, Cormack GC. Misconceptions regarding the cervico-humeral flap. Br J Plast Surg 1983;36:60–3.

5. Pallua N, Machens HG, Rennekampff O, et al. The fasciocutaneous supraclavicular artery island flap for releasing post burn mentosternal contractures. Plast Reconstr Surg 1997;99(7):1878–84.

6. Di Benedetto G, Aquinati A, Pierangeli M, et al. From the "charretera" to the supraclavicular fascial island flap: revisitation and further evolution of a controversial flap. Plast Reconstr Surg 2005;115(1):70–6.

7. Chan JW, Wong C, Ward K, et al. Three- and four-dimensional computed tomographic angiography studies of the supraclavicular artery island flap. Plast Reconstr Surg 2010;125:525–31.

8. Pallua N, Noah EM. The tunneled supraclavicular island flap: an optimized technique for head and neck reconstruction. Plast Reconstr Surg 2000;105(3): 842–52.

9. Sands TT, Martin JB, Simms E, et al. Supraclavicular Artery Island flap innervation: anatomical studies and clinical implications. J Plast Reconstr Aesthet Surg 2012;65:68–71.

10. Su T, Pirgousis P, Fernandes RP. Versatility of supraclavicular Artery Island Flap in Head and Neck Reconstruction of Vessel-Depleted and Difficult Necks. J Oral Maxillofac Surg 2013;71(3): 622–7.

11. Chiu ES, Liu PH, Baratelli R, et al. Circumferential pharyngoesophageal reconstruction with a supraclavicular Artery Island Flap. Plast Reconstr Surg 2010;125:161–6.

12. Epps MT, Cannon CL, Wright MJ, et al. Aesthetic restoration of parotidectomy contour deformity using supraclavicular Artery Island Flap. Plast Reconstr Surg 2011;127(5):1925–31.

13. Pointer DT Jr, Friedlander PL, Amedee RG, et al. Infratemporal fossa reconstruction following total auriculectomy: an alternative flap option. J Plast Reconstr Aesthet Surg 2010;63:e615–8.

14. Moustoukas M, Chan JW, Friedlander PL, et al. Sternal wound coverage using the supraclavicular artery island flap. Plast Reconstr Surg 2012; 129(3):e585–6.

15. Anand AG, Tran EJ, Hasney CP, et al. Oropharyngeal reconstruction using the supraclavicular Artery Island flap: a new flap alternative. Plast Reconstr Surg 2012;129(2):438–41.

16. Chiu ES, Liu PH, Friedlander PL. Supraclavicular Artery Island flap for head and neck oncologic reconstruction: indications, complications and outcomes. Plast Reconstr Surg 2009;124(1):1–9.

17. Conley J. Use of composite flaps containing bone for major repairs in the head and neck. Plast Reconstr Surg 1972;49:522–6.

18. Panje WR. The Island (lateral) trapezius flap. Presented at the Third International Symposium of Plastic and Reconstructive Surgery. New Orleans, April 29–May 4, 1978.

19. Demergasso F. The lateral trapezius flap. Presented at the Third International Symposium of Plastic and Reconstructive Surgery. New Orleans, April 29–May 4, 1978.

20. Mathes SJ, Nahai F. Clinical atlas of muscle and musculocutaneous flaps. St Louis (MO): Mosby; 1979. p. 396.

21. Baek S, Biller HF, Krespi YP, et al. The lower trapezius island myocutaneous flap. Ann Plast Surg 1980;5:108.

22. Taylor GI, Palmer JH. The vascular territories (angiosomes) of the body: experimental study and clinical applications. Br J Plast Surg 1987;40:113–41.

23. Chen WL, Deng YF, Peng JS, et al. Extended Vertical lower trapezius island myocutaneous flap for reconstruction of cranio-maxillofacial defects. Int J Oral Maxillofac Surg 2007;36:165–70.

24. Aviv JE, Urken ML, Lawson W, et al. The superior trapezius myocutaneous flap in head and neck reconstruction. Arch Otolaryngol Head Neck Surg 1992;118:702–6.

25. Ugurlu K, Ozcelik D, Huthut I, et al. Extended vertical trapezius myocutaneous flap in head and neck

reconstruction as a salvage procedure. Plast Reconstr Surg 2004;114:339–50.

26. Chen WL, Yang ZH, Zhang DM, et al. Reconstruction of major full cheek defects with combined extensive pedicled supraclavicular fasciocutaneous island flaps and extended vertical lower Trapezius Island myocutaneous flaps after tumor ablation of advanced oral cancer. J Oral Maxillofac Surg 2012;70:1224–31.

Pectoralis Major Myocutaneous Flap

 CrossMark

Ketan Patel, DDS, PhD[a],*, Diana Jee-Hyun Lyu, DDS[b], Deepak Kademani, DMD, MD[a]

KEYWORDS

- Pectoralis major • Myocutaneous • Surgical flaps • Pedicled flaps • Soft tissue reconstruction

KEY POINTS

- The pectoralis major myocutaneous flap is a widely used pedicled flap in oral and maxillofacial reconstruction, both in replacing tissue loss in avulsive trauma-related and ablative tumor-related defects.
- The pectoralis major myocutaneous flap is favored for its ability to graft a large volume of vascularized muscle with minimal risk of necrosis.
- The thoracoacromial artery and its venae comitantes are the major vessels supplying this flap.
- The major complication associated with this pedicled flap is usually the loss of the skin paddle caused by possible shearing of the perforators during surgery.
- Pedicled pectoralis major myocutaneous flaps should continue to be used appropriately in soft tissue reconstruction as a salvage flap after the loss of a free flap or even considered for patients who have severe comorbidities and are not candidates for a free flap.

INTRODUCTION

Despite the advent of vascularized free tissue grafts, the pectoralis major myocutaneous (PMMC) flap remains a widely used pedicled flap for reconstruction of soft tissue defects in the oral and maxillofacial region. PMMC flaps were originally developed in 1947 for the reconstruction of cardiothoracic tissue defects.[1,2] Ariyan[3] reported the first use of the PMMC flaps in head and neck reconstruction in 1979. Before the PMMC flap, surgeons were using deltopectoral flaps and other local flaps near the head and neck, which did not provide a great bulk of muscle or vasculature.[4] The success of this flap has been recognized, and surgeons began to use the PMMC flap more routinely in head and neck reconstruction. Green and colleagues[5] later described the use of the PMMC flap for reconstruction of mandible using part of the sternum. Ariyan and Cuono[6] further utilized a constchondral segment with a PMMC flap for mandibular segmental reconstructions after ablative defects. The use of double skin paddles for reconstruction of both intraoral and skin defects simultaneously mainly for through and through defects was described thereafter by Ord and Avery.[7]

There has been a gradual shift of the utilization of PMMC pedicled flaps with the current advancements in the successful development of vascularized free flaps. Currently, PMMC flaps are considered a salvage mechanism after failure of a free vascularized flap or used as the reconstructive option for patients who are considered poor candidates for free flaps. In addition, they can be used as chimeric flaps with a free vascularized flap in the reconstruction of gross head and neck defects. This review discusses the PMMC flap for reconstruction of the oral and maxillofacial region, from preoperative considerations and anatomy to surgical technique and possible complications. Advantages and disadvantages for such flaps are also discussed.

The authors have nothing to disclose.
[a] Oral/Head and Neck Oncologic Surgery, Department of Oral and Maxillofacial Surgery, North Memorial Medical Center, 3300 Oakdale Avenue North, Minneapolis, MN 55422, USA; [b] Division of Oral and Maxillofacial Surgery, University of Minnesota, 515 Delaware Street Southeast, Minneapolis, MN 55455, USA
* Corresponding author.
E-mail address: Ketan.Patel@northmemorial.com

Oral Maxillofacial Surg Clin N Am 26 (2014) 421–426
http://dx.doi.org/10.1016/j.coms.2014.05.010
1042-3699/14/$ – see front matter © 2014 Elsevier Inc. All rights reserved.

PREOPERATIVE CONSIDERATIONS

An ideal PMMC flap should include a thorough evaluation of patients and treatment plan, considering aspects that are vital to the success of the flap. These considerations include an ideal treatment sequence, the arc of rotation of the flap, the size of the defect, the color match of the skin donor site to the graft site, and the potential complications of such a procedure.

Treatment Sequence

The source of the original tissue defect should be considered in the sequencing of the PMMC flap. The PMMC is considered a workhouse flap for head and neck reconstruction. Common indications include patients that require salvage head and neck reconstruction after failed microvascular free tissue transfer or in patients that are unwilling or unable because of medical comorbidities to undergo free tissue transfer.

Arc of Rotation of the Flap

The arch of rotation is an important consideration and provides an estimate of the length of the pedicle to be used and also the possible design of the skin paddle. The arc of rotation extends in an oblique fashion from the lateral head of the clavicle to the xiphoid process. The skin paddle, if desired, should be placed in the inferior two-thirds of the incision line to capture the fourth to sixth internal mammary perforators. The arc of rotation can be increased by dissecting off the pectoralis muscle from the humeral head. This humeral head dissection, in turn, increases the effective length of the pedicle. The size of the defect should coincide with the length and width of the skin paddle. The skin color of the chest is not a good match; however, in the realm of salvage surgery or trauma, it is not considered to be much of an issue to patients.

Potential Contraindications

The PMMC flap is the most referenced regional pedicle flap in head and neck reconstructive surgery[8–10] because of the simple graft technique, reliable vascular supply, adequate arc of rotation, and versatility. With increased utilization of vascularized free flaps, PMMC flaps are used as salvage flaps and, therefore, are opted in a circumstance of limited possibilities. Still, it should be noted that certain patients are contraindicated for such flaps. Morbidly obese patients are contraindicated, as they could have a nonviable skin paddle and too much soft tissue bulk to allow for functional reconstruction.[9] Other groups of patients contraindicated for PMMC flaps are those who are congenitally missing the pectoralis muscle, as patients with Poland syndrome. The patients' records should be carefully examined, as patients with previous trauma or surgery to the chest wall could compromise the vasculature to the muscle leading to a poor source of donor tissue. Additionally, patients with vocations requiring full range of motion in their shoulders and arms should be considered with caution, as the PMMC flap harvest could lead to a functional reduction in the movement of the shoulder.

SURGICAL ANATOMY

The pectoralis is a large fan-shaped muscle that covers the anterior chest wall. Its origins are divided into a cephalad (clavicular) portion that attaches to the medial one-third of the clavicle, a central (sternal) portion that arises from the sternum and the first 6 ribs, and a caudal (abdominal) portion that arises from the aponeurosis of the external oblique muscle portion. Each of these divisions has its own vascular and motor supply source. The muscle converges to form a tendon that attaches to the greater tubercle of the humerus and forms the axillary fold.

Laterally, the pectoralis major is closely associated with the medial aspect of the deltoid muscle, forming the deltopectoral groove, which consistently contains the cephalic vein. A layer of deep cervical fascia surrounds the superior surface of the pectoralis major. The inferior surface is separated from the pectoralis minor by the clavipectoral fascia. The clavicopectoral fascia extends cephalad to insert into the inferior aspect of the clavicle, splitting just before its insertion to surround the subclavian muscle.

The blood supply to this muscle includes the pectoral branch of the thoracoacromial artery, the lateral thoracic artery, the superior thoracic artery and the intercostal artery (**Fig. 1**).[11] The pectoralis artery supplies the pectoralis major and arises from the thoracoacromial artery, which, in turn, originates from the second portion of the axillary artery. The lateral thoracic artery, although it is not thought to contribute significantly to the blood supply of the muscle, is often sacrificed to improve the arch of rotation of the muscle. Both arteries are accompanied by their respective venae comitantes.

The tendinous insertion of the pectoralis major on the greater tubercle of the humerus is sacrificed completely to improve the arc of rotation and to increase the effective length of the pedicle. The pectoralis major and overlying skin is supplied by the internal mammary perforators, which anastomose with the thoracoacromial artery branches. Thus

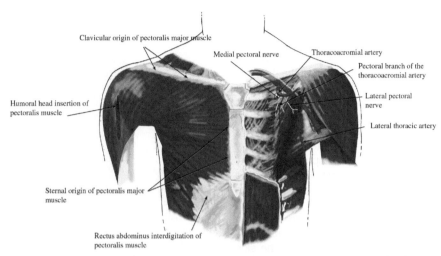

Fig. 1. Arterial supply to the pectoralis major muscle. The blood supply to this muscle includes the pectoral branch of the thoracoacromial artery, lateral thoracic artery, the superior thoracic artery and the intercostal artery. The latter two are not shown in the diagram. (*From* Cordova SW, Bailey JS, Terezides AG. Pectoralis major myocutaneous flap reconstruction of the mandible. Atlas Oral Maxillofac Surg Clin North Am 2006;14(2):171–8; with permission.)

the medial aspect of the muscle is the most reliable area on which to design a skin paddle. Inferiorly, the skin overlying the muscle adjacent to the inferior rectus is supplied by the superior epigastric artery and is the least reliable for skin transfer. The total skin territory of the pectoralis major is almost 400 cm², although it is rare to require such a large skin paddle for a head and neck reconstruction.

Motor innervation to the muscle is supplied by the medial (C5–C7) and lateral (C8-T1) pectoral nerves. The neurovascular bundles pass through the clavipectoral fascia en route to the deep surface of the muscle. The function of the pectoralis major is to adduct and medially rotate the arm.

SURGICAL TECHNIQUE OF THE PMMC FLAP

The first intervention needed before any surgical reconstruction using a PMMC flap is to establish an adequate airway. Oral intubation can be used when a PMMC flap is being performed in isolation. However, if patients are undergoing an extirpation of a primary head and neck tumor with dissection in conjunction with the PMMC flap, then a nasal intubation or a surgical airway is required. A shoulder roll should be placed to allow for optimal neck extension. The endotracheal tube should be secured to allow manipulation of the neck. The use of a tracheostomy should be highly considered when performing this flap because of edema that could be experienced in the postoperative setting.

The incision site should be delineated with a surgical marker, and the skin paddle length and width should correlate to the size of the defect in the head and neck region (**Fig. 2**). Before the incision, the site should be marked and infiltrated with local anesthetic with the vasoconstrictor. The skin paddles that are used are based on the perforators, and usually the goal would be to capture the perforating vessels during the harvest. Adjunctive measures to localize the perforators could include a Doppler or SPY Intraoperative Imaging System for Graft Assessment by LifeCell Corporation (Bridgewater, NJ). The SPY system can also be used at the end of the procedure to ensure good vascularity to the skin paddle.

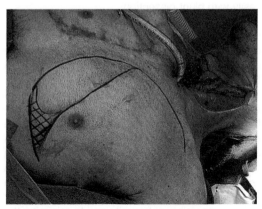

Fig. 2. Incision design of the PMMC flap. The incision site should be delineated with a surgical marker, and the skin paddle length and width should correlate to the size of the defect in the head and neck region.

The clavicle and the lateral border of the sternum are outlined. The vascular pedicle runs vertically along a line drawn from the acromion to the xyphoid process. The skin paddle should be marked on the inferomedial portion of the flap corresponding to the size of the defect. Make a curving C-shaped incision to encompass the skin paddle and allow the breast and skin to be elevated off the chest wall. This incision allows for the preservation of vessels (internal mammary perforators) for a deltopectoral flap in case of any vascular compromise of the pedicle or when the deltopectoral flap is needed as an adjunctive measure.

A No. 10 blade knife can be used to create an incision through the skin and subcutaneous tissue down to the pectoralis fascia encircling the skin paddle. Once the muscle is identified, the inferolateral aspect of the muscle flap is identified and the plane between the pectoralis major and the minor is entered and bluntly dissected. To prevent shearing of the perforators, the skin paddle can be sutured to the pectoralis muscle flap. A broad-based flap is usually harvested to ensure good capture of the perforating vessels to the pectoralis muscle flap.

Dissection is then performed medially on the lateral aspect of the sternum, maintaining a submuscular plane of dissection to the clavicle. Internal mammary perforators are usually encountered between the second and fourth intercostal spaces and need to be identified and clipped to prevent bleeding. This plane should be carefully dissected to prevent inadvertent entry or bleeding into the chest cavity.

As the pectoralis flap is advanced cephalad, the plane of dissection between the major and minor is encountered along the clavipectoral fascia. The plane is relatively avascular and can be opened easily with blunt dissection.

The vascular pedicle is located on the on the upper lateral portion of the flap. The pectoral branch of the thoracoacromial artery can be seen on the deep surface of the pectoralis major and medial to the pectoralis minor (**Fig. 3**).

The muscle divides laterally as it courses toward the humeral insertion. The lateral and medial pectoral nerves along with the lateral vascular pedicle are sacrificed to allow for a greater arc of rotation and to avoid flap contraction with subsequent arm movement. The transection of the pectoral nerves leads to atrophy of the flap that is beneficial in head and neck defects, especially if gross contour defects are visible extraorally and to minimize the torsion/head pull of the flap.

Once the flap is elevated, a broad tunnel is created in the subcutaneous plane to allow the

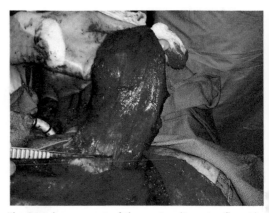

Fig. 3. Advancement of the pectoralis major flap. The pectoral branch of the thoracoacromial artery can be seen on the deep surface of the pectoralis major and medial to the pectoralis minor.

flap to be passed through into the neck. Typically, 3 to 4 fingerbreadths of space are needed to ensure that the pedicle is not compressed or compromised (**Fig. 4**). The flap is subsequently tunneled through the subcutaneous plane created with the skin paddle oriented to prevent torqueing of the pedicle (**Fig. 5**).

Once the flap skin paddle is sutured in place, drains are placed into the donor site in a dependent fashion. The donor site is closed primarily; however, if a large skin paddle is used, then a skin graft needs to be placed over the exposed muscle. The site is closed in a layer fashion with 3-0 vicryl sutures after dependent drains are placed and secured with 2-0 nylon sutures. Staples or nylon sutures can be used to close the skin (**Fig. 6**).

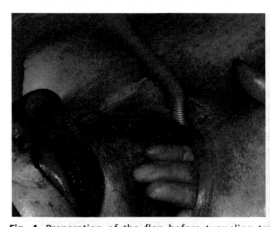

Fig. 4. Preparation of the flap before tunneling to graft site. Once the flap is elevated, a broad tunnel, with 3 to 4 fingerbreadths of space, is created in the subcutaneous plane to allow the flap to be passed through into the neck.

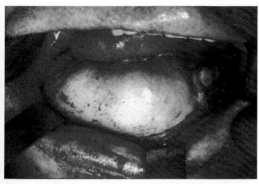

Fig. 5. Inset of flap. The flap is subsequently tunneled through the subcutaneous plane created with the skin paddle oriented to prevent torqueing of the pedicle.

DISCUSSION

With the continuing development and success of the vascularized free flaps, the PMMC flap has taken a secondary role in oral and maxillofacial reconstruction. Still, this does not deviate from the fact that the PMMC flap is a reliable and practical option for soft tissue reconstruction of defects in the oral cavity and face. Historically, evidence-based data have shown success of these PMMC flaps in both trauma and/or tumor-related ablative defects.

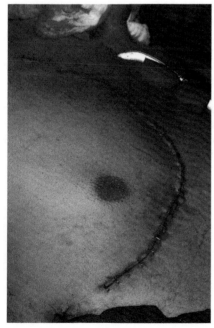

Fig. 6. Donor site closure. The donor site is closed primarily in layers with 3-0 vicryl sutures; however, if a large skin paddle is used, then a skin graft needs to be placed over the exposed muscle. Staples or nylon sutures can be used to close the skin.

As previously discussed, the main indication for the use of the PMMC flap is currently for closure of head and neck defects, including oral cavity, oropharyngeal, pharyngoesophageal, and skull-base defects. It may be used to close an orocutaneous fistula, cover an exposed carotid artery, add bulk to a radical neck dissection site, or restore complex defects with inner and outer epithelial linings. If the muscle flap is used to cover intraoral defects, the muscular surface mucosalizes even without the use of a skin paddle. In patients with severe comorbidities or patients only planned for palliative surgery, these flaps can be used as an alternative to free vascularized flaps for closure of head and neck defects.

The most common complication associated with the PMMC flap is partial or total flap necrosis during the development of the flap. Shah and colleagues[10] found multiple correlated factors that led to the failure of the pectoralis muscle flap. Patients who are greater than 70 years of age, female, and/or nomographic overweight were more likely at risk to develop complications during the development of the flap. The study also noted that poor flap outcomes were associated with patients who have albumin levels less than 4 g/dL; with use of the flap for oral cavity reconstruction after a major glossectomy; and with the presence of systemic diseases, such as diabetes mellitus, hypertension, atherosclerotic heart disease, peripheral vascular disease, renal failure, and collagen vascular disease. The main complications noted were wound infection, fistula formation, and wound dehiscence; these were increased in irradiated patients.

Also, the surgeon should take precautions during the procedure to prevent further risks for developing complications. Larger skin paddles lead to a greater capture of vessel perforators leading to decreased loss of the skin paddle compared with smaller skin paddles that lead to vascular insufficiency. In addition, suturing of the skin paddle to the muscle prevents shearing of the perforators and, therefore, prevents loss of the skin paddle. Carlson[12] discusses the importance of considering the use of the entire muscle to capture a more complete blood supply for better perfusion. Judicious use of the electrocautery should be used, as excessive use can lead to coagulation of the vessels and compromising the vascular pedicle through retrograde thrombosis. Incorporation of the lateral thoracic artery is important for flap viability, particularly if a distal skin paddle is incorporated into the flap. Makiguchi and colleagues[13] found that although the lateral thoracic artery only supplies 6.6% of the mass of the flap, the artery is connected directly to the other branches supplying the muscle, calling the flap "supercharged" by the lateral thoracic artery.

SUMMARY

Historically, the PMMC flap has been referred to as the workhorse in oral and maxillofacial reconstruction, both in replacing tissue loss in avulsive trauma-related and ablative tumor-related defects. Because of its ability to graft a large volume of vascularized muscle without a high risk of necrosis, the PMMC flap was favored for a great percentage of soft tissue reconstruction before the development and success of vascularized free flaps. For the success of these flaps, it is important to consider examining patients in great detail to maximize the benefits and reduce complications, such as planning the arc of rotation and planning a well-sequenced treatment. There were many factors related to possible complications and negative outcomes related to PMMC flaps, some preoperatively based on patients' demographic and medical history and others related to the technique and anatomy dissected during the procedure. One of these main structures determining vitality is the lateral thoracic artery, which has been found to be contributory to the success of the flap through both its central and its branches. Even with vascularized free flaps being preferred for major soft tissue reconstruction, pedicled PMMC flaps should continue to be used appropriately in soft tissue reconstruction as a salvage flap after the loss of a free flap or even considered for patients who have severe comorbidities and are not candidates for a free flap.

REFERENCES

1. Pickrell KL, Baker HM, Collins JP. Reconstructive surgery of the chest wall. Surg Gynecol Obstet 1947;84:465–76.

2. Hueston JT, McConchie IH. A compound pectoral flap. Aust N Z J Surg 1968;38:61–3.

3. Ariyan S. The pectoralis major myocutaneous flap: a versatile flap for reconstruction in the head and neck. Plast Reconstr Surg 1979;63:73–81.

4. Withers EH, Franklin JD, Madden JJ, et al. Pectoralis major musculocutaneous flap: a new flap in head and neck reconstruction. Am J Surg 1979;138: 537–43.

5. Green MF, Gibson JR, Bryson JR, et al. A one-stage correction of mandibular defects using a aplit sternum, pectoralis major osteo-cutaneous transfer. Br J Plast Surg 1981;34:11.

6. Cuono CB, Ariyan S. Immediate reconstruction of a composite mandibular defect with a regional osteo-myocutaneous flap. Plastic and Reconstr Surg 1980;65:477.

7. Ord RA, Avery BS. Side-by-side double paddle pectoralis major flap for cheek defects. Br J Oral Maxillofac Surg 1989;27:177.

8. Ossoff RH, Wurster CF, Berktold RE, et al. Complications after pectoralis major myocutaneous flap reconstruction of head and neck defects. Arch Otolaryngol 1983;109:812–4.

9. Kroll SS, Goeppert H, Jones M, et al. Analysis of complications in 168 pectoralis major myocutaneous flaps used for head and neck reconstruction. Ann Plast Surg 1990;25:93–7.

10. Shah JP, Haribhakti V, Loree TR, et al. Complications of the pectoralis major myocutaneous flap in head and neck reconstruction. Am J Surg 1990;160: 352–5.

11. Cordova SW, Bailey JS, Terezides AG. Pectoralis major myocutaneous flap reconstruction of the mandible. Atlas Oral Maxillofacial Surg Clin N Am 2006;14:171–8.

12. Carlson ER. Pectoralis major myocutaneous flap Oral Maxillofac Surg Clin North Am 2003;15 565–75.

13. Makiguchi T, Yokoo S, Miyazaki H, et al. Supercharged pectoralis major musculocutaneous flap J Craniofac Surg 2013;24(2):e179–82.

The Pedicled Latissimus Dorsi Myocutaneous Flap in Head and Neck Reconstruction

Hui Shan Ong, BDS, MD, Tong Ji, DDS, MD, PhD,
Chen Ping Zhang, DDS, MD, PhD*

KEYWORDS

- Latissimus dorsi myocutaneous flap • Thoracodorsal artery flap • Pedicled flap • Reconstruction

KEY POINTS

- The latissimus dorsi myocutaneous flap (LDMF) is a reliable pedicle that provides broad soft tissue coverage with minimal donor site morbidity.
- The LDMF has favorable skin color and texture match with the recipient sites.
- A pedicled LDMF (PLDMF) is indicated when there is depletion of neck vessels and is usually applied in cases of salvage surgery.
- The LDMF's primary vascular pedicle (thoracodorsal arterial system) will not be hindered by previous head and neck cancer treatment (eg, radical neck dissection and radiation).

INTRODUCTION

The latissimus dorsi myocutaneous flap (LDMF) is a great armamentarium for head and neck reconstructive surgery. Although the LDMF has long been described in the literature (since 1896) for chest wall reconstruction, the first head and neck application was not published until 1978, by Quillen and colleagues.[1] The flap provides broad soft tissue coverage with minimal donor site morbidity. Watson[2] was the first to report the success of transferring the LDMF as a free vascularized flap. With the current high success rate of microvascular surgery, and increased versatility in flap designs, the LDMF has been used most often as a free microvascular flap rather than a pedicled flap. The indications for a pedicled latissimus dorsi myocutaneous flap (PLDMF) can be limited; however, when the clinical situation is called for, it can become a valuable armamentarium for any reconstructive surgeon. The common indications for PLDMF are in cases of salvage surgery or in patients with depleted neck vessels. When compared with other salvage regional flaps (**Table 1**), such as using the pectoralis major myocutaneous flap (PMMF), the PLDMF has the advantages of broader soft tissue availability, less donor site morbidity, and less noticeable donor site scarring. The current review will describe the perioperative issues related to PLDMF in head and neck reconstruction.

PREOPERATIVE CONSIDERATIONS

For most head and neck reconstructions, the PLDMF is not the primary choice. Its major use in

All authors have read and approved the article. All authors abide by the ethical protocol and certified fidelity of this article.

Conflict of Interest: None.

Financial Disclosure: Not applicable.

Department of Oral Maxillofacial-Head & Neck Oncology, Shanghai Ninth People's Hospital, Shanghai Jiao Tong University, 639 Zhi Zao Ju Road, Shanghai 200011, China

* Corresponding author.

E-mail addresses: zhagchenping@gmail.com; zhang.chenping@hotmail.com

Table 1
Comparing of regional flaps in head and neck reconstruction

	PMMF	LDMF	Trapezius
Artery	Thoracoacromial artery	Thoracodorsal artery	Dorsal scapular artery
Anatomic anomalies	Not important	No	Sometimes
Ease of harvesting	Easy	Easy	Moderate
Patient position	Supine	Lateral decubitus	Lateral decubitus
Arc of rotation	Medium	Long	Medium
Versatility of soft tissue design	+	+++	++
Amount of soft tissue	+	+++	++
Contour	Moderately thick	Moderately thick	Thin
Success rate (%)	>90[3]	80–90[4–7]	84[8]
Donor site morbidity	Limited	Minimal	Possible shoulder drop

Abbreviations: LDMF, latissimus dorsi myocutaneous flap; PMMF, pectoralis major myocutaneous flap.

head and neck reconstruction is indicated when free vascularized surgery cannot be performed. Examples include

- Salvage surgery for failed free vascularized flap.
- Patients with depleted neck vessels.

These indications are similar to those in the PMMF procedure. Although these 2 flaps share similar indications, the PLDMF has several advantages that make it a good treatment alternative[9]:

- Largest soft tissue flap that can be harvested in the body.
- Versatility in soft tissue design.
- Donor site skin is hairless, with comparable color match to that in the head and neck region.
- Donor scar is less noticeable.
- Longer arc of rotation.
- Breast or chest wall alteration is minimal.

However, with all of these benefits, the PLDMF remains relatively unpopular with reconstructive surgeons. The major reason for its unpopularity may due to its disadvantages[9]:

- Inability to perform ablative and reconstructive surgery simultaneously (except in cases when recipient site is located in posterior neck or scalp).
- Requires position change for flap harvesting.
- Long vascular pedicle coursing through the axilla and neck may be more vulnerable to neck infection and positional change.
- Risk of injury to brachial plexus[10]

- Increased rate of minor complications (prolonged wound drainage and seroma formation).[11]

There are relatively few contraindications in PLDMF harvesting. Patients who have had previous trauma or axillary surgery (history of breast cancer) are poor candidates for the PLDMF. It is also relatively contraindicated for patients in whom significant upper-arm strength is obligated for employment, sports (skiing), and daily activities (paraplegic).[9]

REGIONAL ANATOMY

The latissimus dorsi is a fanlike muscle with an origin located in the spinous processes of the lower 6 thoracic vertebrae, lumbar vertebrae, sacral vertebrae, and dorsal iliac crest, via thoracolumbar fascia and the external oblique muscle. The muscle fibers pass laterally and are cephalized; then, they insert between the teres major and pectoralis muscles at the humerus. Together with the teres major, it forms the posterior axillary fold.[12–14]

The primary function of the latissimus dorsi is to adduct, extend, and internally rotate the arm ("posterior push" motion). Sacrificing this muscle can lead to the weakening of upper extremity strength. This can create an impact on athletes (swimmers, skiers, or boxers) who require significant upper arm strength. Patients who have neuromuscular disabilities (paraplegic or poliomyelitis) can also be impacted due to the inability to perform functions such as walking with crutches or bed-to-wheelchair transfers.[9]

Otherwise, for most typical patients, the harvesting of the LDMF has minimal impact on normal daily activity.

NEUROVASCULAR ANATOMY

The latissimus dorsi muscle is a class V[15] muscle with a dominant pedicle (thoracodorsal artery and vein) and secondary blood supply (posterior intercostal perforators). The neurovascular system is consistent, with very few anomalies that never interfere with the flap harvesting process. Ninety-five percent of the thoracodorsal arterial branches originate from the subscapular artery, with merely 5% originating directly from the axillary artery.[12–14,16] The dominant pedicle includes the thoracodorsal artery and concomitant vein arising from the subscapular vessels, after the branching of the circumflex scapular vessels. The thoracodorsal pedicle travels in the cephalocaudal direction under the surface of the latissimus dorsi muscle, with a distance of 1.5 to 3.0 cm from the anterior muscle rim, and it typically gives off 1 to 3 branches to the serratus anterior muscle and a branch of the teres major muscle[12–14,16] before entering the muscular hilum at a length that varies between 6.0 and 16.5 cm (average 9.0 cm).[9]

After entering the muscle, the pedicle divides into 2 distinct branches:

- Descending branch: running parallel to the anterior border of the muscle.
- Transverse branch: running parallel to the proximal muscle rim.

This neurovascular anatomy is persistent in 36.0%[17] to 94.5%[18] of all patients. There are multiple branches arising from both the transverse and vertical branches, which subsequently form a dense vascular communications network. The highest density of perforators is along the anterior (lateral) border of the muscle, notably, the upper two-thirds of the muscle.[12–14,16] The lowest density area is the caudal medial part; therefore, the blood supply will be critical and the risk of thrombosis will be higher if skin paddles are to be designed here.

The secondary nondominant blood supply arises from the segmental perforating branches from the intercostal and lumbar arteries. Fundamentally, these vessels enter the deep surface of the muscle, near the posterior midline, and are responsible for the perfusion of the inferior and medial latissimus dorsi. These vessels, however, are prone to disruption during flap harvesting; thereby, the viability of the flap can be compromised.

SURGICAL DEVELOPMENT OF THE PEDICLED LATISSIMUS DORSI MYOCUTANEOUS FLAP
Patient Positioning

The patient is placed in a lateral decubitus position. The head and neck must be carefully supported to prevent impingement of the brachial plexus by the clavicle. The contralateral axilla is padded; however, the ipsilateral arm is supported in an abducted position and included in the operating field that was draped with a sterile stockinette.

Because a change in patient position is required, it is appropriate to change gowns, gloves, and surgical instruments after the oral, head, and neck recipient site preparation. This is to avoid contamination of the clean surgical field with oral bacteria (clean contaminated wound). It is always required to redrape the back after the development of a recipient tissue bed and change in the patient's position.

Flap Design

Surface anatomy
PLDMF harvesting begins with the identification of the surgical landmarks. Important surface landmarks include the following (**Fig. 1**):

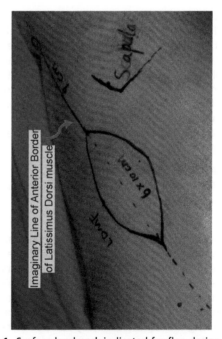

Fig. 1. Surface landmark indicated for flap design. An imaginary line was draw from mid axillary fold to posterior superior iliac spine, this is reliable in predicting the location of anterior rim of latissimus dorsi muscle. Skin paddle shall not be designed too far anteriorly beyond the latissimus dorsi muscle, anterior extension shall be limited to a maximum of 2 cm. Skin paddle shall not be designed above the scapula tip.

- Anterior border of the latissimus dorsi
- Scapular tip
- Mid axillary fold
- Posterior superior iliac spine

The anterior rim of the latissimus dorsi muscle can be located by pinch palpation, and then marked. However, pinch palpation can be difficult in obese subjects. Alternatively, the anterior border of the muscle can be predicted over an imaginary line from the mid axillary groove to the posterior superior iliac spine. It is approximately 8 cm below the midpoint of the axilla, along this imaginary line, where the vascular pedicle enters the undersurface of the latissimus dorsi.

A fusiform-shaped skin paddle is usually designed along the imaginary line. Ideally, the skin paddle should be located over the proximal two-thirds of the latissimus dorsi muscle (primary angiosome); however, the exact location of this skin paddle is dictated by the size of the defect and the arc of rotation. In practice, surgical gauze, placed along the imaginary line and rotated around the anterior axillary fold, can be used to predict the adequacy of rotation. It is acceptable (if needed) to extend the skin paddle a few centimeters lateral to the anterior edge of the muscle to incorporate more cutaneous tissue.

Arc of rotation of the flap

The PLDMF has a long vascular pedicle that can reach as far as the skull vertex. Common reconstructive defects include the oral cavity, pharynx, facial skin, and scalp. When compared with the other 2 pedicled regional flaps (PMMF and trapezius flaps), the PLDMF provides more extended coverage (**Fig. 2**).

The arc of rotation for the PLDMF is limited by several factors:

- Proximal vessel dissection
- Tunneling methods: subcutaneous tunnel versus interpectoral tunnel
- Location of skin paddle

Neck and floor of the mouth defects can be easily reached with a conventional PLDMF design. However, when the defect is cephalic to the maxillary region, dissection proceeds proximally to subscapular artery; sacrificing the circumflex scapular artery can therefore enhance the arc of rotation. Designing the flap more distally can also increase cephalic coverage.

SURGICAL PROCEDURE

PLDMF harvesting is relatively straightforward. The sequence of dissection can be easily broken down into the following steps:

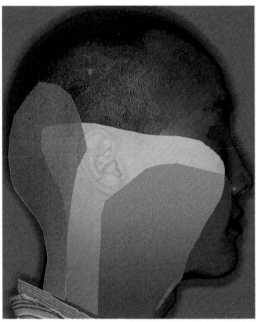

Fig. 2. Color coding indicates the maximal coverage area of different regional flaps: green, trapezius myocutaneous flap; orange, overlapping of latissimus dorsi and pectoral major myocutaneous flaps; red, PMMF; yellow, LDMF.

- Initial incision
- Vascular pedicle identification
- Skin paddle development
- Muscular incision
- Axillary dissection
- Mobilization
- Flap tunneling

Initial Incision

Flap raising begins with an initial skin incision down to the muscle fibers, following the imaginary line and along the anterior border of the skin paddle. The anterior border of the muscle rim can be clearly exposed and separated from the underlying fatty tissue in the lateral to medial direction. This dissection plane is relatively bloodless.

Pedicle Identification

Along this anterior incision, a branch of thoracodorsal artery running anteriorly and supplying the serratus anterior muscle can be appreciated. Dissection along this serratus branch proximally can help to identify the thoracodorsal artery (3–4 cm distal to the serratus branch). Alternatively, the thoracodorsal artery also can be readily located by palpating for its pulse underneath the proximal muscle rim (2 cm medial to the anterior rim of the latissimus dorsi) (**Fig. 3**).

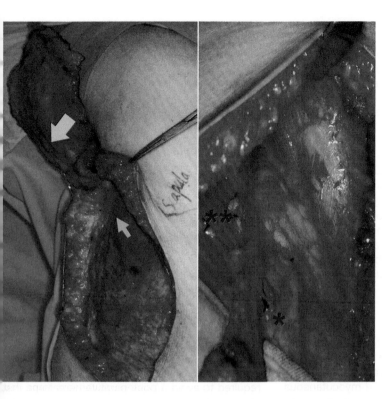

Fig. 3. The PLDMF was raised; the green arrow indicates TDA (thoracodorsal artery with concomitant veins) running parallel to flap longitudinal axis before entering hilum. The blue arrow indicates anterior serratus distal branches before entering the anterior serratus muscle. Dissection of pedicle/TDA proceeded proximally into axilla space, anterior serratus branches (*double asterisk*) and scapular angle branch (*asterisk*) were ligated to increase the arc of rotation of the PLDMF.

Skin Paddle Development

Once the vascular hilum can be observed on the undersurface of the muscle, an incision is made circumferentially around the posteromedial portion of the skin paddle. This incision is made to the level of the fascia overlying the muscle. Before the muscle incision, anchorage sutures are used to secure the skin paddle to the muscle. This step is particularly important in patients with thick subcutaneous tissue. Different tags (lengths of suture) should be used between the anterior and posterior borders, because later, this will be helpful in flap orientation during flap transposition and insertion.

Muscular Incision

Working from the inferior to superior direction, muscle fibers are transected along the inferior pole and medial aspect of the flap. It is prudent to constantly look after the safety of the vascular pedicle running on the undersurface of the flap. This part of the dissection can be facilitated with the use of ultrasonic scissors (Harmonic [Synergy Blade, Ethicon US, Cincinnati, OH, USA]). As the dissection proceeds proximally, branches of thoracodorsal artery (transverse branch to the latissimus dorsi muscle and to the serratus and teres major muscles, angular branch to the scapular tip) must be ligated to fully mobilize the flap.

Axillary Dissection

Following the thoracodorsal artery to the axilla, care should be taken to identify the circumflex scapular and subscapular vessels. This part of the dissection can be facilitated with an assistant abducting and retracting the arm. Care must be taken not to hyperabduct the arm so as to avoid brachial plexus injury. During pedicle dissection, a thin cuff of tissue around the pedicles should be preserved. Fatty loose tissue around the pedicle provides a cushion effect and helps to identify twisting of the pedicle.

For most defects in the lower face and the neck, a PLDMF can reach without sacrificing the circumflex scapular vessel. The preservation of this vessel helps prevent twisting, kinking, or torsion of these long pedicles during delivery; however, if the defect is located midface or superiorly, transaction of the circumflex scapular vessels is required to improve the arc of rotation.[17]

Careful inspection over the thoracodorsal pedicle is a prerequisite, the thoracodorsal nerve is transected if there is a potential of nerve compression over the vascular pedicle. However, the long thoracic nerve to the serratus anterior muscle should be not be intruded and must be preserved.

Mobilization

For the flap to be fully mobilized, the humeral tendon of the latissimus dorsi muscle should be skeletonized. However, it may be wise to wait until the tunnel preparation and wound closure of the back is completed before completing this step. A delay in cutting the humeral tendon helps keep the pedicle safe from inadvertent intraoperative traction, compression, or an injury that might compromise the blood supply, especially in a large flap.

Tunneling

The last step of the procedure is to create a tunnel for flap delivery (**Fig. 4**). There are 2 methods for creating a tunnel: (1) interpectoral tunnel and (2) subcutaneous tunnel. Each method carries its own advantages and disadvantages (**Box 1**, **Table 2**). In most cases, the subcutaneous tunnel is the preferred method because of its ease of development and because it is less likely to impinge the pedicle.

Interpectoral tunnel

The tunnel is formed by blunt dissection (from lateral extending medially) from the anterior axilla to the neck between the pectoralis major and minor muscles. The latissimus dorsi myocutaneous flap will be entering the tunnel and running medially to the thoracoacromial pedicle, reaching the clavipectoral fascia underneath the pectoralis major muscle. A skin incision parallel and inferior to the clavicle is required. The clavicle head portion of the pectoralis major muscle is transected to create an exit pathway for the pedicled flap. This

> **Box 1**
> **Methods to increase the arc of rotation of PLDMF for head and neck reconstruction**
>
> *Methods to increase arc of rotation*
> - Ligation of circumflex scapular artery
> - Interpectoral tunneling
> - Design the skin paddle caudally along the anterior border of the latissimus dorsi

path should be wide enough to accommodate the operator's hand freely between the axilla and neck. When tension is appreciated, several maneuvers can be done:

- Separate the pectoralis minor from its insertion to the coronoid process.
- Acromial branch of the thoracoacromial vessel can be ligated and transected to avoid interference.
- Trimming of the proximal latissimus muscle.

Before flap delivery, meticulous hemostasis is required to avoid a postoperative hematoma that may, inadvertently, compromise the vascular pedicle. After delivery, the vasculature of the pedicle should be checked to ensure that it is free of tension.

Subcutaneous tunnel

The dissection of the subcutaneous tunnel is straightforward at the subcutaneous tissue layer, especially if pectoralis flap has been used. The PLDMF is rotated 180° and passed through the tunnel, reaching the defect region. However, if the cicatricial of the previous surgery is anticipated to cause stress over the pedicle, an incision can be made over the previous scar. As the PLDMF is rotated, the muscular part will be resting over the chest after transposition of flap through the tunnel and resting over the defect region. By now, the pedicle will be protected by muscle and facing downward (ribs) and the latissimus dorsi muscle is facing upward. Chest skin can be sutured to the latissimus dorsi without tension and leaving part of the muscular surface exposed. The exposed muscular surface can be covered with split thickness skin grafting.

POSTOPERATIVE MANAGEMENT

The donor site defect can be closed primarily with generous undermining in the surrounding tissue. Usually, a skin paddle of less than 8 cm in width can be closed without the need for skin grafting.

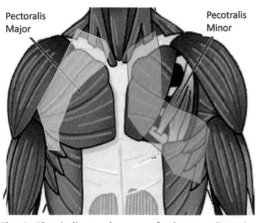

Pectoralis Major

Pecotralis Minor

Fig. 4. Blue indicates the area of subpectoralis major muscle undermining in preparing an interpectoral tunnel; this undermining procedure was performed between the enveloping fascia of pectoralis muscles, which is almost a bloodless field if the thoracoacromial blood vessels remain intact. Yellow indicates area of subcutaneous undermining in preparing a subcutaneous tunnel.

Table 2
Tunneling techniques comparison

	Subcutaneous	Interpectoral
Advantages	Ease of dissection Limited compression within the tunnel	Increase arc of rotation
Disadvantages	Shorter arc of rotation	Difficult dissection Compression from the pectoralis muscle Possible trauma to the thoracoacromial artery

Negative pressure drains should be placed for wound closure, and the drains are removed when there is less than 20 mL of fluid in 24 hours. Skin sutures or clips are left in for 7 to 10 days. If tension is appreciated, the sutures should be left in for a longer period of time. Excessive shoulder movement should be discouraged to prevent wound dehiscence. Gradual return to normal shoulder function can begin on postoperative day 7.[9]

COMPLICATIONS

Intraoperative Complications

Because PLDMF harvesting is relatively straightforward, very few intraoperative complications have been reported. Some of the foreseeable complications may relate to (1) unnecessary injury to the serratus anterior or long thoracic nerve during dissection, or (2) brachial plexus injury from inadequate cushion support during patient positioning. If the surgeon encounters an inadequate arc of rotation, this is most likely due to poor treatment planning.

It is important to note that modifications of the latissimus dorsi myocutaneous flap published in the literature are usually designed for a free flap. These modifications are, in many cases, not applicable in its pedicle form when reconstructing head and neck defects. Most of the modifications (harvesting with serratus anterior, or with scapular angle or separate flap based on the transverse branch of thoracodorsal artery) can greatly limit the arc of rotation.

Postoperative Complications

Donor site

Seroma formation is a relatively common complication seen in PLDMF harvesting. Hayden and colleagues[4] report a 30% rate of seroma formation. However, most seromas can be resolved with Penrose drainage, serial needle aspiration, and compression dressing.

Functional deficits of the shoulder and arm from the loss of the latissimus dorsi muscle are estimated to average 7% in most patients.[9] Fortunately, most deficits can be alleviated with postoperative physical therapy. For the most part, patients do not experience any difficulty in performing normal daily activities; however, for those who require the use of crutches, the effect can be noticeable. The absence of the latissimus dorsi muscle also can lead to pelvic instability in paraplegic patients.

FLAP SUCCESS RATE

Although the PLDMF has long been described (since the late 1970s), there are few studies reporting its success rate. In general consensus, PLDMF has a lower success rate than that in PMMF, and an average success rate of 85% has been reported in the literature (**Table 3**).[4–7] Most flap failures are related to poor vascularity in the distal aspect of the flap, and excessive tension developing in the tunnel (especially in patients with previous neck dissection and radiation). Hayden and colleagues[4] reported a higher success rate compared with previous studies, and the investigators credit their higher success rate to the modified "otter tail" design. Unlike the conventional skin

Table 3
Incidence of PLDMF necrosis

Study	Number	Flap Necrosis (Partial)
Barton et al,[5] 1983	60	6.7% (0%)
Chowdhury et al,[6] 1988	60	10% (11%)
Haughey & Fredrickson,[7] 1991	19	11% (0%)
Davis et al,[11] 1992	90	3% (5%)
Hayden et al,[4] 2000	68	1% (9%)

island paddle, the "otter tail" has a long skin paddle that provides additional perfusion to the distal skin paddle via the dermal, subdermal, and fasciocutaneous system.

SUMMARY

The PLDMF is not the first-line reconstructive option for most clinicians; however, when treating salvage patients or those with depleted neck vessels, PLDMF provides a valuable armamentarium. Unlike PMMF or the lower island trapezius flap, PLDMF has greater versatility in soft tissue design and a longer arc of rotation. These advantages are of great importance in managing advanced reconstructive cases.

REFERENCES

1. Quillen CG, Shearin JC, Georgiade NG. Use of the latissimus dorsi myocutaneous island flap for reconstruction in head and neck area. Plast Reconstr Surg 1978;63:664–70.

2. Watson JS. The use of the latissimus dorsi island flap for intra-oral reconstruction. Br J Plast Surg 1982;35:408–12.

3. Carlson ER. Pectoralis major myocutaneous flap. Oral Maxillofac Surg Clin North Am 2003;15: 565–75.

4. Hayden RE, Kirby SD, Deschler DG. Technical modifications of the latissimus dorsi pedicled flap to increase versatility and viability. Laryngoscope 2000; 110:352–7.

5. Barton FE Jr, Spicer TE, Byrd HS. Head and neck reconstruction with the latissimus dorsi myocutaneous flap: anatomic observations and report of 60 cases. Plast Reconstr Surg 1983;71: 199–204.

6. Chowdhury CR, McLean NR, Harrop-Griffiths K, et al. The repair of defects in the head and neck region with the latissimus dorsi myocutaneous flap. J Laryngol Otol 1988;102:1127–32.

7. Haughey BH, Fredrickson JM. The latissimus dorsi donor site. Current use in head and neck reconstruction. Arch Otolarngol Head Neck Surg 1991; 117:1129–34.

8. Netterville JL, Panje WR, Maves MD. The trapezius myocutaneous flap. Arch Otolarngol Head Neck Surg 1987;113:271–81.

9. Germann G, Ohlbauer M. Latissimus dorsi flap. In: Wei FC, Mardini S, editors. Flap and reconstructive surgery. Philaedelphia: Saunders Inc; 2009. p. 287–319.

10. Sabatier RE, Bakamjian VY. Transaxillary latissimus dorsi flap reconstruction in head and neck cancer. Limitations and refinements in 56 cases. Am J Surg 1985;150:427–34.

11. Davis JF, Garth RJ, Breach NM. The latissimus dorsi flap in head and neck reconstructive surgery: a review of 121 procedures. Clin Otolaryngol 1992;17: 487–90.

12. Saijo M. The vascular territories of the dorsal trunk: a reappraisal for potential flap donor sites. Br J Plast Surg 1978;31:200–4.

13. Aviv JE, Urken ML, Vickery C, et al. The combined latissimus dorsi-scapular free flap in head and neck reconstruction. Arch Otolaryngol Head Neck Surg 1991;117:1242–50.

14. Bartlett SP, May JW Jr, Yaremchuk MJ. The latissimus dorsi muscle: a fresh cadaver study of the primary neurovascular pedicle. Plast Reconstr Surg 1981;67:631–5.

15. Mathes SJ, Nahai F. Classification of the vascular anatomy of muscles: experimental and clinical correlation. Plast Reconstr Surg 1981;67:177–87.

16. Bostwick J 3rd. Latissimus dorsi flap: current applications. Ann Plast Surg 1982;9:377–80.

17. Rowsell AR, Davis DM, Eisenberg N, et al. The anatomy of the subscapular-thoracodorsal arterial system: study of 100 cadaver dissections. Br J Plast Surg 1984;37:574–6.

18. Har-El G, Bhaya M, Sundaram K. Latissimus dorsi myocutaneous flap for secondary head and neck reconstruction. Am J Otolaryngol 1999;20:287–93.

Index

Note: Page numbers of article titles are in **boldface** type.

oralmaxsurgery.theclinics.com

Printed and bound by CPI Group (UK) Ltd, Croydon, CR0 4YY

03/10/2024

01040375-0014